MIND DIET COOKBOOK

FOR SENIORS OVER 60

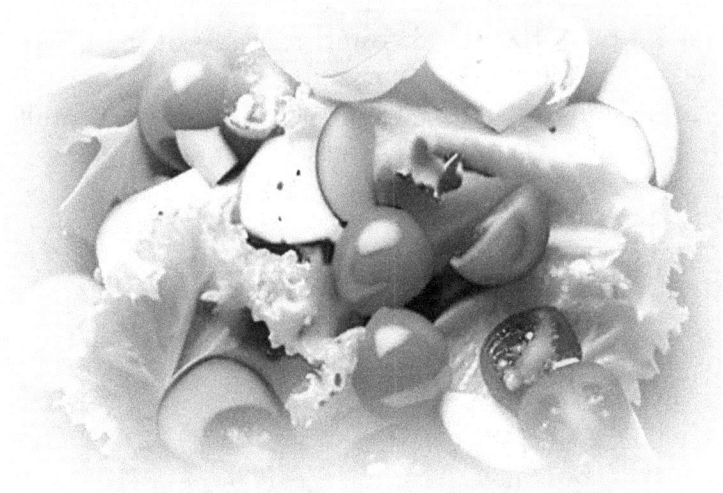

1500 Days Quick, Easy, And Delicious Recipes To Help
Improve Brain Function, Fight Memory Disorder,
Alzheimer's, and Dementia

Dr. Charlene Alexander

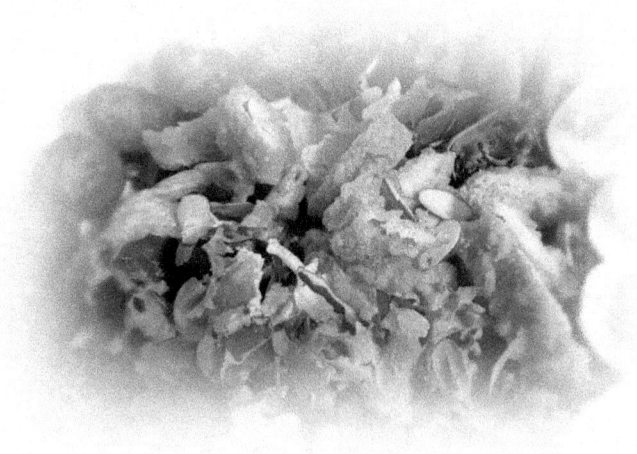

TABLE OF CONTENTS

INTRODUCTION 7

CHAPTER 1: Understanding the MIND Diet 9

Foods to Limit 11
The Benefits of the MIND Diet for Seniors 12
Portion Control for Seniors 14
Strategies for Effective Portion Control 16
Practical Tips for Meal Preparation 17

CHAPTER 2: Breakfasts 18

Blueberry Almond Oatmeal 18
Spinach and Feta Omlet 19
Avocado Toast with Poached Egg 20
Whole Grain Waffles with Mixed Berries 21
Greek Yogurt Parfait 22
Vegetable Frittata 23
Nutty Banana Smoothie 25
Salmon and Avocado Bagel 26
Quinoa Breakfast Bowl 27
Kale and Mushroom Breakfast Sauté 28

CHAPTER 3: Lunches 30

Mediterranean Quinoa Salad 30
Grilled Salmon with Steamed Greens 31

Lentil Soup with Whole Grain Bread 32

Turkey and Avocado Wrap 34

Spinach and Strawberry Salad with Walnuts 35

Baked Sweet Potato with Black Bean Salsa 36

Broccoli and Almond Stir-Fry 38

Tuna Salad Stuffed Tomatoes 39

Roasted Vegetable and Hummus Pita Pockets 40

Barley and Roasted Beet Salad 42

CHAPTER 4: Dinners 44

Baked Cod with Lemon and Dill over Quinoa 44

Roasted Chicken with Sweet Potatoes and Brussels Sprouts ... 45

Vegetable Lentil Stew with Whole Grain Rolls 46

Grilled Vegetable and Bean Tacos with Avocado Salsa 48

Whole Wheat Pasta Primavera with Seasonal Vegetables 50

Stuffed Bell Peppers with Brown Rice and Turkey 51

Baked Eggplant Parmesan with a Side Salad 53

Salmon Quinoa Patties with Steamed Asparagus 55

Turkey Meatballs in Tomato Sauce with Steamed Broccoli 56

Spinach and Mushroom Stuffed Chicken Breast with Wild Rice
.... 58

CHAPTER 5: Snacks and Sides 61

Carrot and Celery Sticks with Hummus 61

Greek Yogurt with Blueberries and a Drizzle of Honey 61

Sliced Apple with Almond Butter 62

Whole Grain Crackers with Avocado Mash 62

Roasted Chickpeas with Garlic and Herbs.............................. 63

Walnut and Date Energy Balls 64

Cucumber Rounds Topped with Smoked Salmon and Cream Cheese 66

Baked Sweet Potato Fries with Rosemary 67

Steamed Edamame with Sea Salt.................................... 68

Kale Chips Baked 69

CHAPTER 6: Desserts 71

Baked Apples with Cinnamon and Walnuts.......................... 71

Blueberry Almond Chia Pudding.................................... 72

Dark Chocolate-Dipped Strawberries 73

Whole Wheat Banana Bread with Flaxseeds 74

Mixed Berry and Yogurt Parfait..................................... 76

Almond and Date Energy Bites 77

Peach and Berry Cobbler with Oat Topping 78

Avocado Chocolate Mousse.. 80

Carrot Cake Muffins with Whole Wheat Flour...................... 81

Grilled Pineapple with Honey and Greek Yogurt 82

CHAPTER 7: Smoothies and Beverages 84

Blueberry Walnut Smoothie... 84

Strawberry Oat Heart-Healthy Smoothie............................ 84

Green Tea and Citrus Boost 85

Turmeric Ginger Zinger 86

Avocado and Kale Smoothie... 87

Berry and Beet Detox Smoothie 88

Almond Butter and Banana Protein Shake 89

Pomegranate and Cherry Antioxidant Drink.......................... 90

Cucumber Mint Refresh.. 91

Golden Milk Latte.. 92

CHAPTER 8: SOUPS 93

Lentil and Vegetable Soup 93

Tomato Basil Soup with Whole whole-grain Croutons 94

White Bean and Kale Minestrone 96

Carrot Ginger Soup with Turmeric 97

Quinoa and Black Bean Chili 99

Mushroom Barley Soup 100

Split Pea Soup with Thyme.. 101

Butternut Squash and Apple Soup 102

Broccoli Almond Soup.. 104

Chickpea and Spinach Stew.. 105

CONCLUSION 107

28-DAY MEAL PLAN.. 108

INTRODUCTION

Welcome to a culinary voyage designed especially for the golden years, where nutrition meets taste to nourish both body and mind. This cookbook is more than just a collection of recipes; it's a guide to embracing a lifestyle that can brighten your days and sharpen your wits. As we age, our dietary needs evolve, and this book aims to cater to those changes, focusing particularly on the MIND diet, a plan celebrated for its positive impact on brain health.

The MIND diet, short for Mediterranean-DASH Intervention for Neurodegenerative Delay, is a harmonious blend of the Mediterranean and DASH diets, both acclaimed for their health benefits. It's specifically tailored to reduce the risk of dementia and cognitive decline, making it an ideal choice for those over 60. By emphasizing foods like leafy greens, berries, whole grains, olive oil, and fish, the MIND diet offers a delicious approach to eating that supports brain health.

Let me share a story that underscores the power of the MIND diet. Imagine Sarah, a vibrant 65-year-old with a passion for gardening and a love for her grandchildren. Lately, Sarah noticed her memory wasn't as sharp as it used to be, making her worry about missing out on precious moments with her family. That's when she discovered the MIND diet and decided to give it a try. Within months, Sarah felt a noticeable difference. Not only did she enjoy the flavors and variety of the meals, but she also found herself more engaged during family game nights, recalling stories with clarity and laughing more freely.

Sarah's experience is just one of many that illustrate how the MIND diet can transform lives. This cookbook is your gateway to a similar transformation. Whether you're cooking for yourself, a loved one, or friends, these recipes are designed to be simple, nutritious, and, above all, delightful.

CHAPTER 1: Understanding the MIND Diet

The MIND diet, an acronym for the Mediterranean-DASH Intervention for Neurodegenerative Delay, is a nutritional framework designed to reduce the risk of dementia and decline in brain health. It is a hybrid of two well-established diets: the Mediterranean diet, known for its heart-healthy and anti-inflammatory benefits, and the DASH (Dietary Approaches to Stop Hypertension) diet, developed to combat high blood pressure. The MIND diet stands out for its focus on specific foods that research has linked to improved cognitive function and a lower risk of neurodegenerative diseases.

Core Components of the MIND Diet

The MIND diet emphasizes the following food groups, encouraging frequent consumption for their brain-boosting properties:

Green Leafy Vegetables: Such as spinach, kale, and collards, are recommended to be eaten at least six times a week for their high levels of vitamins and minerals.

Other Vegetables: Encouraged daily, these provide essential nutrients and fiber, contributing to overall health.

Berries: Particularly blueberries and strawberries, are singled out for their antioxidant properties and are recommended at least twice a week.

Nuts: A source of healthy fats, protein, and fiber, nuts are recommended as snacks five times a week.

Whole Grains: At least three servings a day are encouraged, providing essential nutrients and fiber.

Fish: Especially fatty fish rich in omega-3 fatty acids, recommended at least once a week.

Poultry: Like chicken or turkey, suggested twice a week as a healthier protein alternative to red meat.

Beans: Including lentils and other legumes, recommended at least three times a week for their protein and fiber.

Olive Oil: Recommended as the main cooking oil, rich in monounsaturated fats and antioxidants.

Wine: Moderate consumption, particularly red wine, is suggested (up to one glass per day), due to compounds like resveratrol that may benefit brain health.

Foods to Limit

The MIND diet also identifies foods that are potentially harmful to brain health and recommends limiting their intake:

Red Meats: Suggested less than four times a week.

Butter and Margarine: Advised to use less than a tablespoon daily, encouraging olive oil as a healthier fat.

Cheese: Recommended less than once a week due to high saturated fat content.

Sweets and Pastries: Limited due to sugar and refined flour, which can impact cognitive health.

Fried and Fast Food: Suggested less than once a week due to unhealthy fats and preservatives.

Benefits and Flexibility

The MIND diet's strength lies in its combination of foods rich in antioxidants, vitamins, and healthy fats, which contribute to reducing oxidative stress and inflammation, factors associated with cognitive decline. Research has shown that even moderate adherence to the MIND diet can offer protective benefits against Alzheimer's and other forms of dementia.

One of the appealing aspects of the MIND diet is its flexibility. Unlike stricter diets, it allows individuals to benefit from it without the need for perfect adherence. This makes it more sustainable over the long term and adaptable to various lifestyles and dietary preferences.

The Benefits of the MIND Diet for Seniors

The MIND diet offers numerous benefits for seniors, particularly in promoting brain health and reducing the risk of neurodegenerative diseases such as Alzheimer's. This diet is not only about what you eat; it's about nurturing your mind with every meal. Here are some key benefits of the MIND diet for seniors:

Enhanced Cognitive Function

The MIND diet emphasizes nutrients that are vital for brain health, including omega-3 fatty acids from fish, antioxidants from berries and vegetables, and healthy fats from nuts and olive oil. These nutrients support neuron health and cognitive functions, potentially slowing cognitive decline associated with aging.

Reduced Risk of Alzheimer's and Dementia

Research suggests that strict adherence to the MIND diet can significantly lower the risk of Alzheimer's disease. Even moderate adherence can offer protective benefits, making it a compelling choice for anyone looking to protect their brain health as they age.

Heart Health Benefits

The MIND diet borrows heavily from the Mediterranean and DASH diets, both known for their cardiovascular benefits. Promoting whole grains, lean proteins, and healthy fats, supports heart health, reducing the risk of hypertension, stroke, and heart disease, which are common concerns for seniors.

Antioxidant-Rich

Foods recommended in the MIND diet, such as berries, leafy greens, and nuts, are high in antioxidants. These compounds combat oxidative stress and inflammation in the body, which are linked to chronic diseases and aging. Antioxidants can help protect cells from damage, supporting overall health and longevity.

Weight Management

The MIND diet focuses on natural, whole foods and limits high-calorie, processed foods. This can naturally lead to healthier weight management, which is crucial for mobility, joint health, and chronic disease prevention in older adults.

Easy to Follow and Flexible

Unlike some restrictive diets, the MIND diet offers flexibility, allowing individuals to benefit from it without needing to adhere perfectly. This adaptability makes it easier for seniors to incorporate the diet into their lifestyles, enhancing long-term sustainability.

Improved Nutritional Intake

By focusing on a variety of nutrient-dense foods, the MIND diet ensures that seniors receive a broad spectrum of vitamins, minerals, and other nutrients essential for maintaining health and vitality.

Social and Mental Wellbeing

Cooking and enjoying meals from the MIND diet can also have social benefits, encouraging family meals and social gatherings centered around healthy, delicious food. This can boost mental well-being and provide a sense of community and belonging.

Incorporating the principles of the MIND diet into daily life can offer seniors a pathway to not only maintaining but also enhancing their cognitive and physical health. It's about creating a diet that feeds the mind as much as the body, ensuring that the later years are enjoyed with clarity, vitality, and joy.

Portion Control for Seniors

Portion control is a crucial aspect of healthy eating for seniors, impacting not only weight management but also overall health and well-being. As metabolism naturally slows with age, and activity levels may decrease, seniors often require fewer calories. However, the need for nutrient-dense foods becomes even more important to maintain energy, support cognitive function, and prevent chronic diseases. Here's how portion control can benefit seniors and some strategies to implement it effectively:

Benefits of Portion Control for Seniors

Weight Management: Proper portion sizes help maintain a healthy weight, reducing the risk of obesity-related conditions such as type 2 diabetes, heart disease, and joint issues.

Nutrient Intake: By focusing on portion sizes, seniors can ensure they're getting a balanced diet rich in essential nutrients without overeating.

Digestive Health: Smaller, well-balanced meals can be easier to digest, reducing the risk of gastrointestinal discomfort and improving nutrient absorption.

Blood Sugar Regulation: Controlled portions, especially carbohydrates, can help maintain stable blood sugar levels, crucial for seniors with or at risk of diabetes.

Energy Levels: Regular, appropriately sized meals and snacks can help maintain steady energy levels throughout the day.

Strategies for Effective Portion Control

Use Smaller Plates: Downsizing from a standard dinner plate to a salad plate can visually make portions appear larger, leading to satisfaction with smaller amounts of food.

Read Labels: Understanding serving sizes on nutritional labels can help seniors gauge how much of a packaged food is considered a reasonable portion.

Meal Planning: Preparing and possibly pre-measuring meals can prevent overeating and ensure a balanced intake of nutrients.

Mindful Eating: Encouraging seniors to eat slowly and without distractions (like TV) can help increase awareness of hunger and fullness cues, preventing overeating.

Hydration: Drinking water before meals can help control appetite, as thirst is often mistaken for hunger.

Vegetable Focus: Filling half the plate with vegetables before adding proteins or grains can ensure a nutrient-rich meal with lower calorie density.

Share Meals: Especially when dining out, where portions can be generous, sharing a meal can prevent overeating and reduce waste.

Practical Tips for Meal Preparation

Pre-portion Snacks: Dividing snacks into individual portions ahead of time can prevent mindless overeating from larger containers.

Batch Cooking: Preparing meals in bulk and dividing them into single-serving containers can simplify portion control and meal variety throughout the week.

Visual Cues: Familiarizing with visual cues for common portion sizes can be helpful, such as equating a serving of meat to the size of a deck of cards or a serving of grains to a tennis ball.

Implementing these portion control strategies can help seniors enjoy a variety of foods while maintaining their health, energy, and overall quality of life. It's about finding the right balance that sustains the body's needs without overindulgence, ensuring that every meal contributes positively to their well-being.

CHAPTER 2: Breakfasts

Blueberry Almond Oatmeal

Ingredients:

- 1 cup rolled oats
- 2 cups almond milk (unsweetened)
- 1 cup fresh or frozen blueberries
- 2 tablespoons sliced almonds
- 1 tablespoon honey or maple syrup (optional)
- 1/2 teaspoon vanilla extract (optional)
- A pinch of salt

Instructions:

1. In a medium saucepan, bring the almond milk to a low boil. Add a pinch of salt and the rolled oats. Reduce the heat to a simmer.
2. Cook the oats, stirring occasionally, for about 5 minutes, or until the oats have absorbed the milk and reached your desired consistency.
3. Stir in the vanilla extract and half of the blueberries, cooking for an additional minute.

4. Divide the oatmeal into bowls. Top each bowl with the remaining blueberries, sliced almonds, and a drizzle of honey or maple syrup for added sweetness, if desired.

5. Serve warm.

Spinach and Feta Omlet

Ingredients:

- 2 large eggs
- 1 cup fresh spinach, chopped
- 1/4 cup feta cheese, crumbled
- 1 tablespoon olive oil
- Salt and pepper to taste
- Optional: diced tomatoes, onions, or herbs for extra flavor

Instructions:

1. Wash and chop the spinach. If using additional vegetables, prepare them as well.

2. In a bowl, whisk the eggs with salt and pepper until well combined.

3. Heat olive oil in a non-stick skillet over medium heat. Add the spinach (and any other vegetables you're using) and sauté until the spinach is wilted, about 1-2 minutes.

4. Pour the beaten eggs over the spinach. Tilt the pan to ensure the eggs cover the spinach evenly.

5. Sprinkle the crumbled feta cheese over the eggs as they begin to set.

6. Let the eggs cook undisturbed for a few minutes until the edges start to set. With a spatula, gently fold one side of the omelet over the other.

7. Carefully slide the omelet onto a plate. Serve hot.

Avocado Toast with Poached Egg

Ingredients:

- 1 ripe avocado
- 2 slices whole-grain bread
- 2 eggs
- Vinegar (for poaching eggs)
- Salt and pepper to taste
- Optional toppings: red pepper flakes, chia seeds, or a sprinkle of lemon juice

Instructions:

1. Toast the whole-grain bread slices to your liking.

2. Mash the avocado in a bowl and season with salt and pepper. Spread the mashed avocado evenly on the toasted bread slices.

3. Bring a pot of water to a gentle simmer and add a splash of vinegar. Crack each egg into a small bowl and gently slide them

into the simmering water one at a time. Poach for about 3-4 minutes or until the whites are set but the yolks remain runny.

4. Use a slotted spoon to remove the eggs from the water, draining well.

5. Place a poached egg on top of each avocado toast. Season with salt, pepper, and any additional toppings you prefer.

6. Serve immediately, enjoying the creamy texture of the avocado with the richness of the poached egg.

Whole Grain Waffles with Mixed Berries

Ingredients:

- 1 cup whole grain flour (such as whole wheat or oat flour)
- 1 tablespoon baking powder
- 1/4 teaspoon salt
- 1 cup milk (dairy or plant-based)
- 1 egg
- 2 tablespoons olive oil or melted unsalted butter
- 1 tablespoon honey or maple syrup
- 1 teaspoon vanilla extract
- 2 cups mixed berries (blueberries, strawberries, raspberries)
- Optional: yogurt or additional honey/maple syrup for serving

Instructions:

1. Preheat your waffle iron according to the manufacturer's instructions.

2. In a large bowl, whisk together the whole-grain flour, baking powder, and salt.

3. In another bowl, beat the egg and then mix in the milk, olive oil or melted butter, honey or maple syrup, and vanilla extract.

4. Pour the wet ingredients into the dry ingredients and stir until just combined; be careful not to overmix.

5. Cook the waffles according to your waffle iron's instructions, usually pouring about 1/4 cup of batter for each waffle and cooking until golden and crisp.

6. While the waffles are cooking, prepare the mixed berries. If using strawberries, slice them to match the size of the other berries.

7. Serve the waffles hot, topped with the mixed berries. Add a dollop of yogurt or a drizzle of honey or maple syrup if desired.

Greek Yogurt Parfait

Ingredients:

- 2 cups Greek yogurt (plain or vanilla)
- 1 cup granola
- 1 cup mixed berries (such as blueberries, strawberries, raspberries)
- Honey or maple syrup for drizzling (optional)

- A few mint leaves for garnish (optional)

Instructions:

1. If using strawberries, slice them into bite-sized pieces.
2. In serving glasses or bowls, start by layering a spoonful of Greek yogurt at the bottom.
3. Add a layer of granola over the yogurt.
4. Add a layer of mixed berries on top of the granola.
5. Repeat the layers until the glasses or bowls are filled, finishing with a layer of berries on top.
6. Drizzle a little honey or maple syrup over the top for added sweetness, if desired.
7. Garnish with mint leaves for a fresh touch.
8. Serve immediately or refrigerate until ready to serve.

Vegetable Frittata

Ingredients:

- 8 eggs
- 1/2 cup milk
- 1 cup spinach, chopped
- 1/2 cup bell peppers, diced
- 1/2 cup tomatoes, diced
- 1/4 cup onions, diced

- 1/2 cup cheese (feta, cheddar, or goat cheese work well), crumbled or shredded
- 2 tablespoons olive oil
- Salt and pepper to taste
- Optional: herbs such as parsley or basil for garnish

Instructions:

1. Preheat your oven to 375°F (190°C) if your skillet is oven-safe. If not, you'll transfer the frittata to a baking dish before baking.
2. In a large bowl, whisk the eggs and milk together until well combined. Season with salt and pepper.
3. Heat olive oil in a large, oven-safe skillet over medium heat. Sauté onions, bell peppers, and tomatoes until they're soft, about 5 minutes.
4. Add the chopped spinach to the skillet, and cook until just wilted, about 1-2 minutes.
5. Pour the egg mixture over the sautéed vegetables in the skillet, ensuring the ingredients are evenly distributed. Sprinkle the cheese evenly over the top.
6. Cook on the stovetop over medium heat until the edges of the frittata start to set, about 2-3 minutes.
7. Transfer the skillet to the preheated oven (or pour the mixture into a baking dish if your skillet is not oven-safe) and bake for

15-20 minutes, or until the frittata is set and the top is lightly golden.

8. Remove from the oven and let it cool for a few minutes. Slice into wedges and garnish with fresh herbs if desired.

9. Serve warm.

Nutty Banana Smoothie

Ingredients:

- 1 ripe banana
- 1 tablespoon nut butter (almond, peanut, or cashew)
- 1 cup almond milk or milk of choice
- 1/2 cup Greek yogurt (plain or vanilla)
- A handful of spinach leaves (optional for added nutrients)
- 1 tablespoon chia seeds or flaxseeds (optional)
- A handful of ice cubes
- Honey or maple syrup to taste (optional)

Instructions:

1. Peel the banana and break it into chunks.

2. Place the banana chunks, nut butter, almond milk, Greek yogurt, and spinach leaves if using, into a blender.

3. Add the chia seeds or flaxseeds if desired for extra fiber and omega-3s.

4. Add a handful of ice cubes to make the smoothie cold and refreshing.

5. Blend on high until smooth and creamy. Add a bit of honey or maple syrup if you prefer a sweeter smoothie.

6. Pour the smoothie into a glass and enjoy immediately.

Salmon and Avocado Bagel

Ingredients:

- 2 whole grain bagels, halved and toasted
- 4 oz smoked salmon
- 1 ripe avocado
- 1 tablespoon cream cheese or Greek yogurt (for a healthier option)
- 1 teaspoon lemon juice
- Salt and pepper to taste
- Optional: capers, red onion slices, or fresh dill for garnish

Instructions:

1. Halve and toast the bagels to your preferred level of crispiness.

2. In a small bowl, mash the avocado with lemon juice, salt, and pepper until it's creamy but still has some texture.

3. Spread a thin layer of cream cheese or Greek yogurt on each bagel half.

4. Spread the mashed avocado mixture over the cream cheese or yogurt.

5. Arrange slices of smoked salmon on top of the avocado.

6. If desired, add capers, thin slices of red onion, and a sprig of fresh dill for extra flavor and garnish.

7. Season with a little more salt and pepper to taste. Serve immediately.

Quinoa Breakfast Bowl

Ingredients:

- 1 cup cooked quinoa
- 1/2 cup almond milk or milk of choice
- 1/4 teaspoon cinnamon
- 1 apple, diced
- 1/4 cup walnuts, chopped
- 2 tablespoons raisins or dried cranberries
- Honey or maple syrup to taste
- A pinch of salt

Instructions:

1. Warm the cooked quinoa in a pot over medium heat, adding the almond milk to create a creamy consistency.

2. Stir in the cinnamon and a pinch of salt, mixing well.

3. Once the quinoa is warmed through, transfer it to a bowl.

4. Top the quinoa with diced apple, chopped walnuts, and raisins or dried cranberries.

5. Drizzle with honey or maple syrup for a touch of sweetness.

6. Serve warm.

Kale and Mushroom Breakfast Sauté

Ingredients:

- 2 cups kale, chopped and stems removed
- 1 cup mushrooms, sliced
- 2 cloves garlic, minced
- 2 tablespoons olive oil
- 2 eggs (optional, for added protein)
- Salt and pepper to taste
- Optional: grated Parmesan or nutritional yeast for a cheesy flavor

Instructions:

1. Heat the olive oil in a large skillet over medium heat.

2. Add the minced garlic and sauté for about 30 seconds until fragrant.

3. Add the sliced mushrooms to the skillet, seasoning with salt and pepper. Sauté until the mushrooms are golden and tender, about 5-7 minutes.

4. Add the chopped kale to the skillet, stirring frequently until the kale is wilted and tender, about 3-5 minutes.

5. If adding eggs, make two wells in the kale and mushroom mixture and crack an egg into each. Cover the skillet and cook until the eggs are set to your liking.

6. Season the entire dish with additional salt and pepper to taste. If desired, sprinkle with grated Parmesan or nutritional yeast for added flavor.

7. Serve hot.

CHAPTER 3: Lunches

Mediterranean Quinoa Salad

Ingredients:

- 1 cup quinoa
- 2 cups water or vegetable broth
- 1 cup cherry tomatoes, halved
- 1 cucumber, diced
- 1/2 red onion, finely chopped
- 1/2 cup Kalamata olives, halved
- 1/2 cup feta cheese, crumbled
- 1/4 cup fresh parsley, chopped
- 3 tablespoons olive oil
- 2 tablespoons lemon juice
- Salt and pepper to taste

Instructions:

1. Rinse the quinoa under cold water to remove its natural coating, saponin, which can make it taste bitter.
2. In a medium saucepan, combine the quinoa and water (or vegetable broth) and bring to a boil. Reduce the heat to low, cover, and simmer for 15 minutes, or until the quinoa is fluffy and the water is absorbed.

3. Remove from heat and let it stand for 5 minutes, then fluff with a fork and allow to cool.

4. In a large bowl, combine the cooled quinoa, cherry tomatoes, cucumber, red onion, Kalamata olives, feta cheese, and parsley.

5. In a small bowl, whisk together the olive oil, lemon juice, salt, and pepper. Pour the dressing over the salad and toss to combine.

6. Serve chilled or at room temperature. This salad can be stored in the refrigerator for up to 3 days, making it a great make-ahead lunch option.

Grilled Salmon with Steamed Greens

Ingredients:

- 4 salmon fillets (about 6 ounces each)
- 2 tablespoons olive oil
- Salt and pepper to taste
- 1 lemon, sliced
- 4 cups mixed greens (such as spinach, kale, and Swiss chard)
- Optional: garlic, herbs (like dill or parsley), or a sprinkle of lemon zest for extra flavor

Instructions:

1. Preheat the grill to medium-high heat. If using an oven, preheat it to 400°F (200°C) and prepare a baking sheet lined with foil or parchment paper.

2. Brush both sides of the salmon fillets with olive oil and season with salt and pepper. Place a few slices of lemon on top of each fillet.

3. If grilling, place the salmon fillets skin-side down on the grill and cook for 6-8 minutes, or until the salmon is opaque and flakes easily with a fork. If baking, place the fillets on the prepared baking sheet and bake for 12-15 minutes.

4. While the salmon is cooking, steam the mixed greens. You can do this by placing them in a steamer basket over boiling water, covering them, and steaming them for 3-5 minutes, or until the greens are wilted but still vibrant.

5. Serve the grilled or baked salmon on a bed of steamed greens. Garnish with additional lemon slices, fresh herbs, or a sprinkle of lemon zest if desired.

Lentil Soup with Whole Grain Bread

Ingredients:

- 1 cup dried lentils, rinsed and drained
- 1 tablespoon olive oil
- 1 onion, chopped
- 2 carrots, diced
- 2 celery stalks, diced
- 2 garlic cloves, minced
- 1 teaspoon ground cumin

- 1/2 teaspoon ground coriander (optional)
- 4 cups vegetable broth or water
- 1 can (14 oz) diced tomatoes, with juice
- Salt and pepper to taste
- Fresh parsley or cilantro for garnish
- Slices of whole grain bread for serving

Instructions:

1. Heat the olive oil in a large pot over medium heat. Add the chopped onion, carrots, and celery. Sauté until the vegetables are softened, about 5 minutes.
2. Add the minced garlic, ground cumin, and coriander if using, and cook for another minute until fragrant.
3. Stir in the rinsed lentils, vegetable broth, and diced tomatoes with their juice. Season with salt and pepper.
4. Bring the mixture to a boil, then reduce the heat, cover, and simmer for about 25-30 minutes, or until the lentils are tender.
5. If desired, use an immersion blender to partially puree the soup for a thicker consistency, or leave it chunky.
6. Adjust the seasoning if necessary, then ladle the soup into bowls. Garnish with chopped parsley or cilantro.
7. Serve the soup hot, accompanied by slices of hearty whole-grain bread for dipping.

Turkey and Avocado Wrap

Ingredients:

- 2 whole grain tortillas or wraps
- 6 ounces sliced turkey breast (preferably low sodium)
- 1 ripe avocado, sliced
- 1 cup mixed salad greens or baby spinach
- 1/4 cup shredded carrots
- 2 tablespoons hummus or Greek yogurt
- Salt and pepper to taste
- Optional: thin slices of cucumber, tomato, or red onion for extra crunch and flavor

Instructions:

1. Lay out the whole-grain tortillas on a flat surface.
2. Spread a tablespoon of hummus or Greek yogurt on each tortilla. This adds flavor and helps hold the wrap together.
3. Place an even layer of mixed greens or baby spinach on top of the hummus/yogurt.
4. Add the sliced turkey breast over the greens, distributing it evenly across the tortillas.
5. Arrange the avocado slices and shredded carrots on top of the turkey. If using additional vegetables like cucumber, tomato, or red onion, add them now.
6. Season with a little salt and pepper to taste.

7. Carefully roll up each tortilla, tucking in the sides as you go, to form a wrap.

8. Cut the wraps in half diagonally for easier eating, if desired.

9. Serve immediately, or wrap tightly in foil or plastic wrap for a convenient and nutritious lunch on the go.

Spinach and Strawberry Salad with Walnuts

Ingredients:

- 4 cups fresh baby spinach leaves
- 1 cup strawberries, hulled and sliced
- 1/2 cup walnuts, roughly chopped
- 1/4 cup crumbled feta cheese or goat cheese (optional)
- 2 tablespoons balsamic vinegar
- 1 tablespoon olive oil
- 1 teaspoon honey or maple syrup
- Salt and pepper to taste

Instructions:

1. In a large salad bowl, combine the baby spinach leaves and sliced strawberries.

2. In a dry pan over medium heat, lightly toast the walnuts for 2-3 minutes, just until they're aromatic. Be careful not to burn them. Allow them to cool slightly before adding them to the salad.

3. If using, sprinkle the crumbled feta cheese or goat cheese over the salad for added creaminess and flavor.

4. In a small bowl, whisk together the balsamic vinegar, olive oil, and honey or maple syrup to create the dressing. Season with a pinch of salt and pepper to taste.

5. Drizzle the dressing over the salad just before serving and gently toss to ensure all the ingredients are evenly coated.

6. Serve the salad immediately to enjoy the fresh flavors and crisp textures.

Baked Sweet Potato with Black Bean Salsa

Ingredients for Baked Sweet Potato:

- 4 medium sweet potatoes, scrubbed clean
- 1 tablespoon olive oil
- Salt to taste

Ingredients for Black Bean Salsa:

- 1 can (15 oz) black beans, rinsed and drained
- 1/2 cup corn kernels (fresh, frozen and thawed, or canned)
- 1 medium tomato, diced
- 1/4 cup red onion, finely chopped
- 1/4 cup cilantro, chopped
- Juice of 1 lime
- Salt and pepper to taste

- Optional: diced avocado or a dollop of Greek yogurt for topping

Instructions:

1. Preheat the oven to 400°F (200°C). Line a baking sheet with foil or parchment paper for easy cleanup.
2. Prick the sweet potatoes all over with a fork, then rub them with olive oil and sprinkle lightly with salt. Place them on the prepared baking sheet.
3. Bake the sweet potatoes for 45-60 minutes, or until they are tender and a fork can easily pierce through the flesh.
4. While the sweet potatoes are baking, prepare the black bean salsa. In a medium bowl, combine the black beans, corn, diced tomato, red onion, and cilantro. Squeeze the lime juice over the top and season with salt and pepper. Stir to combine everything evenly.
5. Once the sweet potatoes are done, let them cool for a few minutes, then slice them open lengthwise without cutting all the way through.
6. Spoon a generous amount of the black bean salsa into each sweet potato. If desired, top with diced avocado or a dollop of Greek yogurt for extra creaminess.
7. Serve the stuffed sweet potatoes warm, with any extra salsa on the side.

Broccoli and Almond Stir-Fry

Ingredients:

- 4 cups broccoli florets
- 1/2 cup almonds, sliced or whole
- 2 tablespoons olive oil
- 2 garlic cloves, minced
- 1 tablespoon soy sauce (low sodium preferred)
- 1 teaspoon sesame oil
- 1/2 teaspoon ground ginger or 1 tablespoon fresh ginger, grated
- Salt and pepper to taste
- Optional: red pepper flakes for a bit of heat, sesame seeds for garnish

Instructions:

1. Heat a large skillet or wok over medium heat. Add the almonds and toast them lightly until they're golden brown and fragrant, stirring frequently to prevent burning. Remove the almonds from the skillet and set aside.

2. In the same skillet, increase the heat to medium-high and add the olive oil. Once hot, add the broccoli florets and stir-fry for about 4-5 minutes, or until they are bright green and tender-crisp.

3. Add the minced garlic (and red pepper flakes if using) to the broccoli, stirring constantly for about 30 seconds to prevent the garlic from burning.

4. Drizzle the soy sauce, sesame oil, and ginger over the broccoli, stirring to coat the florets evenly in the seasoning. Cook for an additional 1-2 minutes.

5. Return the toasted almonds to the skillet and toss with the broccoli to mix well.

6. Season with salt and pepper to taste, and sprinkle with sesame seeds if desired.

7. Serve hot as a nutritious and flavorful side dish or over a bed of brown rice or quinoa for a complete meal.

Tuna Salad Stuffed Tomatoes

Ingredients:

- 4 large tomatoes
- 1 can (5 oz) tuna in water, drained and flaked
- 1/4 cup celery, finely diced
- 1/4 cup red onion, finely chopped
- 2 tablespoons mayonnaise or Greek yogurt for a healthier option
- 1 tablespoon fresh lemon juice
- 1 tablespoon fresh parsley, chopped
- Salt and pepper to taste
- Optional: a sprinkle of paprika or chopped chives for garnish

Instructions:

1. Slice the tops off the tomatoes and use a spoon to gently scoop out the seeds and inner flesh to create a hollow space. Be careful not to break the skin. Set the hollowed-out tomatoes aside.

2. In a medium bowl, mix the flaked tuna, diced celery, chopped red onion, mayonnaise or Greek yogurt, lemon juice, and chopped parsley. Stir until all the ingredients are well combined. Season with salt and pepper to taste.

3. Spoon the tuna salad mixture into the hollowed-out tomatoes, filling them generously.

4. Garnish the tops with a sprinkle of paprika or chopped chives if desired for added color and flavor.

5. Serve the stuffed tomatoes chilled or at room temperature as a refreshing and protein-packed lunch option.

Roasted Vegetable and Hummus Pita Pockets

Ingredients:

- 2 medium zucchinis, sliced
- 1 red bell pepper, sliced
- 1 yellow bell pepper, sliced
- 1 red onion, sliced
- 2 tablespoons olive oil

- Salt and pepper to taste
- 4 whole grain pita bread rounds
- 1 cup hummus
- Optional: baby spinach leaves, cucumber slices, or feta cheese for added freshness and flavor

Instructions:

1. Preheat the oven to 425°F (220°C). Line a large baking sheet with parchment paper.

2. In a large bowl, toss the sliced zucchini, bell peppers, and red onion with olive oil, salt, and pepper until well coated.

3. Spread the vegetables in a single layer on the prepared baking sheet. Roast in the preheated oven for 20-25 minutes, or until the vegetables are tender and lightly caramelized, stirring halfway through.

4. Warm the pita bread in the oven during the last few minutes of roasting or on a skillet over low heat.

5. Cut the pita bread rounds in half to form pockets. Spread a generous layer of hummus inside each pita pocket.

6. Fill each pita pocket with the roasted vegetables. If desired, add baby spinach, cucumber slices, or crumbled feta cheese for additional flavor and texture.

7. Serve the pita pockets immediately while the vegetables are still warm.

Barley and Roasted Beet Salad

Ingredients:

- 1 cup pearl barley, rinsed
- 3 cups water or vegetable broth
- 4 medium beets, peeled and diced
- 2 tablespoons olive oil, divided
- 1/4 cup balsamic vinegar
- 1 tablespoon honey or maple syrup
- 1/2 cup walnuts, roughly chopped
- 1/2 cup goat cheese, crumbled
- 1/4 cup fresh parsley, chopped
- Salt and pepper to taste

Instructions:

1. Preheat the oven to 400°F (200°C).
2. In a medium saucepan, combine the barley and water (or vegetable broth). Bring to a boil, then reduce heat to low, cover, and simmer for 30-40 minutes, or until the barley is tender and the liquid is absorbed. Allow to cool.
3. Toss the diced beets with 1 tablespoon of olive oil and season with salt and pepper. Spread them out on a baking sheet lined with parchment paper.

4. Roast the beets in the preheated oven for 25-30 minutes or until tender and caramelized, stirring occasionally.

5. In a small bowl, whisk together the remaining olive oil, balsamic vinegar, and honey or maple syrup to create a dressing. Season with salt and pepper to taste.

6. In a large salad bowl, combine the cooked barley, roasted beets, walnuts, and crumbled goat cheese.

7. Drizzle the dressing over the salad and toss gently to combine.

8. Garnish with chopped parsley before serving. This salad can be served warm or at room temperature.

CHAPTER 4: Dinners

Baked Cod with Lemon and Dill over Quinoa

Ingredients:

- 4 cod fillets (about 6 ounces each)
- 2 tablespoons olive oil
- 2 lemons (1 sliced, 1 juiced)
- 2 tablespoons fresh dill, chopped (or 2 teaspoons dried dill)
- Salt and pepper to taste
- 1 cup quinoa
- 2 cups water or vegetable broth

Instructions:

1. Preheat your oven to 400°F (200°C). Line a baking sheet with parchment paper or lightly grease it with olive oil.

2. Rinse the quinoa under cold water until the water runs clear. Combine the quinoa and water (or broth) in a medium saucepan. Bring to a boil, then reduce heat to low, cover, and simmer for 15-20 minutes, or until the quinoa is fluffy and the liquid is absorbed.

3. While the quinoa is cooking, place the cod fillets on the prepared baking sheet. Drizzle with olive oil and lemon juice, then season with salt and pepper.

4. Place lemon slices on top of each fillet and sprinkle with dill.

5. Bake in the preheated oven for 12-15 minutes, or until the cod is opaque and flakes easily with a fork.

6. Fluff the cooked quinoa with a fork and divide it among plates. Top with the baked cod fillets, garnishing with additional dill if desired. Serve immediately.

Roasted Chicken with Sweet Potatoes and Brussels Sprouts

Ingredients:

- 4 chicken breasts (bone-in, skin-on)
- 2 sweet potatoes, peeled and cubed
- 2 cups Brussels sprouts, halved
- 3 tablespoons olive oil
- 1 teaspoon paprika
- 1 teaspoon garlic powder
- Salt and pepper to taste
- Fresh herbs (like thyme or rosemary) for garnish (optional)

Instructions:

1. Preheat your oven to 425°F (220°C).

2. Line a large baking sheet with parchment paper or lightly grease it.

3. In a large bowl, toss the sweet potato cubes and Brussels sprouts with 2 tablespoons of olive oil, salt, and pepper until they are evenly coated.

4. Spread the vegetables in a single layer on one side of the prepared baking sheet, leaving room for the chicken.

5. Rub the remaining olive oil over the chicken breasts and season them with paprika, garlic powder, salt, and pepper.

6. Place the seasoned chicken breasts skin-side up on the other side of the baking sheet.

7. Roast in the preheated oven for 25-30 minutes, or until the chicken is cooked through (reaching an internal temperature of 165°F or 74°C) and the vegetables are tender and caramelized.

8. Let the chicken rest for a few minutes before serving. Garnish with fresh herbs if desired.

9. Serve the roasted chicken alongside the sweet potatoes and Brussels sprouts.

Vegetable Lentil Stew with Whole Grain Rolls

Ingredients for Stew:

- 1 cup dried green or brown lentils, rinsed
- 2 tablespoons olive oil

- 1 onion, chopped
- 2 carrots, diced
- 2 celery stalks, diced
- 2 garlic cloves, minced
- 1 teaspoon dried thyme
- 1/2 teaspoon smoked paprika
- 4 cups vegetable broth
- 1 can (14 oz) diced tomatoes
- 2 cups chopped kale or spinach
- Salt and pepper to taste
- Optional: a splash of red wine vinegar or lemon juice for added brightness

Instructions:

1. Heat the olive oil in a large pot over medium heat. Add the chopped onion, carrots, and celery, cooking until they begin to soften, about 5 minutes.
2. Stir in the minced garlic, dried thyme, and smoked paprika, cooking for another minute until fragrant.
3. Add the rinsed lentils, vegetable broth, and diced tomatoes with their juice to the pot. Season with salt and pepper.
4. Bring the mixture to a boil, then reduce the heat to low, cover, and simmer for about 25-30 minutes, or until the lentils are tender.

5. Stir in the chopped kale or spinach and continue to simmer until the greens have wilted about 5 minutes. Adjust the seasoning as needed.

6. If desired, add a splash of red wine vinegar or lemon juice to the stew before serving to enhance the flavors.

7. Serve the stew hot, accompanied by whole grain rolls for a hearty and nutritious meal.

Grilled Vegetable and Bean Tacos with Avocado Salsa

Ingredients for Tacos:

- 2 zucchinis, sliced lengthwise
- 1 bell pepper, sliced
- 1 red onion, sliced
- 1 can (15 oz) black beans, rinsed and drained
- 2 tablespoons olive oil
- 1 teaspoon ground cumin
- 1/2 teaspoon chili powder
- Salt and pepper to taste
- Whole wheat or corn tortillas

Ingredients for Avocado Salsa:

- 1 ripe avocado, diced
- 1 tomato, diced

- 1/4 cup red onion, finely chopped
- Juice of 1 lime
- 2 tablespoons chopped cilantro
- Salt to taste

Instructions:

1. Preheat your grill or grill pan to medium-high heat.
2. In a large bowl, toss the sliced zucchini, bell pepper, and red onion with olive oil, ground cumin, chili powder, salt, and pepper until well coated.
3. Grill the vegetables, turning occasionally, until they are tender and charred in spots, about 8-10 minutes.
4. Warm the black beans in a small pot over low heat, seasoned with a pinch of cumin, chili powder, and salt.
5. Warm the tortillas on the grill for about 30 seconds on each side until they are pliable and slightly charred.
6. To make the avocado salsa, gently mix the diced avocado, tomato, red onion, lime juice, and chopped cilantro in a bowl. Season with salt to taste.
7. Assemble the tacos by placing a scoop of black beans on each tortilla, topped with grilled vegetables and a spoonful of avocado salsa.
8. Serve the tacos immediately.

Whole Wheat Pasta Primavera with Seasonal Vegetables

Ingredients:

- 8 ounces whole wheat pasta (like spaghetti or penne)
- 2 tablespoons olive oil
- 2 garlic cloves, minced
- 1 cup broccoli florets
- 1 cup asparagus, cut into 1-inch pieces
- 1 medium carrot, julienned
- 1 zucchini, sliced
- 1/2 cup cherry tomatoes, halved
- 1/4 cup peas (fresh or frozen and thawed)
- 1/4 cup low-sodium vegetable broth
- Juice and zest of 1 lemon
- Salt and pepper to taste
- 1/4 cup grated Parmesan cheese
- Fresh basil leaves, for garnish

Instructions:

1. Cook the whole wheat pasta according to package instructions in a large pot of salted boiling water until al dente. Drain and set aside, reserving 1 cup of pasta water.

2. Heat the olive oil in a large skillet over medium heat. Add the minced garlic and sauté for 1 minute until fragrant.

3. Add the broccoli, asparagus, and carrots to the skillet. Cook for about 4-5 minutes, stirring occasionally, until the vegetables start to soften.

4. Stir in the zucchini, cherry tomatoes, and peas. Cook for an additional 2-3 minutes until all the vegetables are tender yet crisp.

5. Pour in the vegetable broth and bring to a simmer. Add the cooked pasta to the skillet, tossing to combine with the vegetables. If the mixture seems dry, add a little reserved pasta water to reach the desired consistency.

6. Stir in the lemon juice and zest, and season with salt and pepper to taste.

7. Serve the pasta primavera sprinkled with grated Parmesan cheese and garnished with fresh basil leaves.

Stuffed Bell Peppers with Brown Rice and Turkey

Ingredients:

- 4 large bell peppers, tops cut off and seeds removed
- 1 cup cooked brown rice
- 1 tablespoon olive oil
- 1/2 pound ground turkey

- 1 onion, chopped

- 2 garlic cloves, minced

- 1 can (14 oz) diced tomatoes, drained

- 1 teaspoon dried oregano

- 1 teaspoon dried basil

- Salt and pepper to taste

- 1/2 cup shredded mozzarella cheese

- Fresh parsley, for garnish

Instructions:

1. Preheat the oven to 375°F (190°C).

2. Blanch the bell peppers by boiling them in water for 5 minutes to soften slightly. Drain and set aside in a baking dish.

3. In a skillet, heat the olive oil over medium heat. Add the ground turkey and cook until browned, breaking it apart with a spoon.

4. Add the chopped onion and minced garlic to the skillet with the turkey. Cook until the onion is translucent.

5. Stir in the cooked brown rice, diced tomatoes, oregano, and basil. Season with salt and pepper. Cook for an additional 5 minutes, allowing the flavors to meld.

6. Spoon the turkey and rice mixture into each blanched bell pepper, packing it tightly.

7. Top each stuffed pepper with shredded mozzarella cheese.

8. Cover the baking dish with foil and bake in the preheated oven for 25-30 minutes. Remove the foil and bake for an additional 5-10 minutes until the cheese is bubbly and golden.

9. Garnish with fresh parsley before serving. Enjoy a comforting and nutritious meal that's perfect for any night of the week.

Baked Eggplant Parmesan with a Side Salad

Ingredients for Eggplant Parmesan:

- 2 medium eggplants, sliced into 1/2-inch rounds
- Salt for drawing out moisture from the eggplant
- 2 cups whole wheat breadcrumbs
- 1 tablespoon Italian seasoning
- 2 eggs, beaten
- 2 cups marinara sauce, low-sodium
- 2 cups shredded mozzarella cheese
- 1/2 cup grated Parmesan cheese
- Fresh basil leaves for garnish

Ingredients for Side Salad:

- 4 cups mixed salad greens
- 1 cup cherry tomatoes, halved
- 1/4 cup thinly sliced red onion
- 2 tablespoons olive oil

- 1 tablespoon balsamic vinegar
- Salt and pepper to taste

Instructions for Eggplant Parmesan:

1. Preheat the oven to 375°F (190°C). Place eggplant slices in a single layer on paper towels and sprinkle both sides with salt. Let sit for 20-30 minutes to draw out moisture, then pat dry.
2. Mix the breadcrumbs with Italian seasoning. Dip each eggplant slice in the beaten eggs, then coat with the breadcrumb mixture. Place on a baking sheet lined with parchment paper.
3. Bake the eggplant slices for 20 minutes, flipping halfway through, until golden and tender.
4. In a baking dish, spread a thin layer of marinara sauce. Layer half of the baked eggplant slices over the sauce, then top with half of the mozzarella and Parmesan cheese. Repeat the layers, finishing with cheese on top.
5. Bake for 25-30 minutes, or until the cheese is melted and bubbly.
6. Garnish with fresh basil leaves before serving.

Instructions for Side Salad:

1. In a large bowl, combine the mixed salad greens, cherry tomatoes, and red onion.
2. Whisk together the olive oil and balsamic vinegar, then season with salt and pepper.
3. Drizzle the dressing over the salad and toss to combine.

4. Serve the salad alongside the baked eggplant Parmesan for a complete and nutritious meal.

Salmon Quinoa Patties with Steamed Asparagus

Ingredients for Salmon Quinoa Patties:

- 1 cup cooked quinoa
- 1 can (14 oz) salmon, drained and flaked
- 2 green onions, finely chopped
- 2 eggs
- 1/4 cup whole wheat breadcrumbs
- 1 tablespoon Dijon mustard
- 1 tablespoon lemon juice
- 2 tablespoons fresh dill, chopped (or 1 teaspoon dried dill)
- Salt and pepper to taste
- Olive oil for cooking

Ingredients for Steamed Asparagus:

- 1 bunch asparagus, trimmed
- Salt and pepper to taste
- Lemon wedges for serving

Instructions for Salmon Quinoa Patties:

1. In a large bowl, combine the cooked quinoa, flaked salmon, green onions, eggs, breadcrumbs, Dijon mustard, lemon juice, and dill. Season with salt and pepper and mix well.

2. Form the mixture into patties, about 3-4 inches in diameter.

3. Heat a little olive oil in a large skillet over medium heat. Cook the patties for 4-5 minutes on each side, or until golden brown and heated through.

Instructions for Steamed Asparagus:

1. Bring a pot of water to a boil and place a steamer basket with the asparagus over the water, ensuring the water doesn't touch the bottom of the basket.

2. Cover and steam the asparagus for 3-5 minutes, or until tender-crisp.

3. Season the asparagus with salt and pepper and serve with lemon wedges on the side.

Turkey Meatballs in Tomato Sauce with Steamed Broccoli

Ingredients for Turkey Meatballs:

- 1 pound ground turkey
- 1/4 cup whole wheat breadcrumbs
- 1/4 cup grated Parmesan cheese

- 1 egg
- 2 garlic cloves, minced
- 1 teaspoon dried oregano
- Salt and pepper to taste
- Ingredients for Tomato Sauce:
- 2 cups low-sodium marinara sauce
- 1 onion, chopped
- 2 garlic cloves, minced
- 1 tablespoon olive oil
- 1 teaspoon dried basil

Ingredients for Steamed Broccoli:

- 1 large head of broccoli, cut into florets
- Salt and pepper to taste
- Lemon wedges for serving

Instructions:

1. Preheat the oven to 375°F (190°C). Line a baking sheet with parchment paper.
2. In a bowl, mix the ground turkey, breadcrumbs, Parmesan, egg, minced garlic, oregano, salt, and pepper until well combined.
3. Form the mixture into 1-inch meatballs and place them on the prepared baking sheet.

4. Bake the meatballs for 20-25 minutes, or until they're cooked through and lightly browned.

5. While the meatballs are baking, heat the olive oil in a large skillet over medium heat. Sauté the chopped onion and minced garlic until softened.

6. Add the marinara sauce and dried basil to the skillet, and bring to a simmer.

7. Once the meatballs are done, add them to the tomato sauce in the skillet, coating them well. Simmer for an additional 10 minutes.

8. Steam the broccoli florets until tender-crisp, about 3-5 minutes. Season with salt and pepper.

9. Serve the turkey meatballs and sauce with a side of steamed broccoli. Garnish with lemon wedges.

Spinach and Mushroom Stuffed Chicken Breast with Wild Rice

Ingredients for Chicken:

- 4 boneless, skinless chicken breasts
- 2 cups fresh spinach, chopped
- 1 cup mushrooms, chopped
- 1/2 cup feta cheese, crumbled
- 2 tablespoons olive oil
- Salt and pepper to taste

Ingredients for Wild Rice:

- 1 cup wild rice blend
- 2 1/2 cups water or low-sodium chicken broth
- Salt to taste

Instructions:

1. Preheat the oven to 375°F (190°C).
2. In a skillet, heat 1 tablespoon of olive oil over medium heat. Sauté the spinach and mushrooms until the spinach is wilted and the mushrooms are soft. Let the mixture cool slightly, then mix in the feta cheese.
3. Cut a pocket into the side of each chicken breast, being careful not to cut all the way through.
4. Stuff each chicken breast with the spinach, mushroom, and feta mixture. Secure the openings with toothpicks if necessary.
5. Season the outside of the chicken breasts with salt and pepper. In the same skillet, heat the remaining olive oil over medium-high heat. Sear the chicken on both sides until golden, about 2-3 minutes per side.
6. Transfer the chicken to a baking dish and bake in the preheated oven for 20-25 minutes, or until the chicken is cooked through and no longer pink inside.

7. While the chicken is baking, rinse the wild rice blend and combine it with water (or chicken broth) in a saucepan. Bring to a boil, then reduce the heat to low, cover, and simmer for 45-50 minutes, or until the rice is tender and the liquid is absorbed. Season with salt to taste.

8. Serve the stuffed chicken breasts with a side of wild rice.

CHAPTER 5: Snacks and Sides

Carrot and Celery Sticks with Hummus

Ingredients:

- 2 large carrots
- 2 large celery stalks
- 1 cup hummus (store-bought or homemade)

Instructions:

1. Wash and peel the carrots. Rinse the celery stalks under cold water to clean them.
2. Cut the carrots and celery into sticks approximately 3 to 4 inches long and 1/2 inch wide, making them easy to dip.
3. Serve the carrot and celery sticks on a plate with a bowl of hummus in the center for dipping.

Greek Yogurt with Blueberries and a Drizzle of Honey

Ingredients:

- 1 cup Greek yogurt (plain, unsweetened)
- 1/2 cup fresh blueberries (you can also use frozen blueberries, thawed)
- 1 tablespoon honey

Instructions:

1. Spoon the Greek yogurt into a serving bowl.
2. Top the yogurt with fresh blueberries, evenly distributing them over the yogurt.
3. Drizzle the honey over the top of the blueberries and yogurt.
4. Mix lightly before eating, if desired, or enjoy the layers of yogurt, blueberries, and honey as they are.

Sliced Apple with Almond Butter

Ingredients:

- 1 large apple (such as Fuji, Gala, or Granny Smith)
- 2-3 tablespoons almond butter

Instructions:

1. Wash the apple thoroughly under running water.
2. Using a sharp knife, core the apple and slice it into thin rounds or wedges, depending on your preference.
3. Spread a layer of almond butter on each apple slice. The amount of almond butter can be adjusted according to taste.
4. Arrange the almond butter-topped apple slices on a plate.

Whole Grain Crackers with Avocado Mash

Ingredients:

- 1 ripe avocado

- 1 tablespoon lime or lemon juice
- Salt and pepper to taste
- A pinch of chili flakes or paprika (optional)
- Whole grain crackers

Instructions:

1. Cut the avocado in half and remove the pit. Scoop out the flesh into a small bowl.
2. Add the lime or lemon juice to the avocado to prevent browning and enhance flavor.
3. Mash the avocado with a fork until it reaches your desired consistency. Some people prefer a smooth mash, while others like it a bit chunky.
4. Season the avocado mash with salt, pepper, and, if desired, a pinch of chili flakes or paprika for a little extra kick.
5. Spread the avocado mash generously onto whole-grain crackers.
6. Serve immediately to enjoy the creamy texture of the avocado with the crunchy whole-grain crackers.

Roasted Chickpeas with Garlic and Herbs

Ingredients:

- 1 can (15 oz) chickpeas, drained, rinsed, and patted dry
- 2 tablespoons olive oil
- 1 teaspoon garlic powder

- 1 teaspoon dried rosemary (or thyme, oregano, or a mix of your favorite herbs)
- Salt and pepper to taste

Instructions:

1. Preheat your oven to 400°F (200°C). Line a baking sheet with parchment paper for easy cleanup.
2. In a bowl, toss the dried chickpeas with olive oil, ensuring they are evenly coated.
3. Sprinkle the garlic powder, dried herbs, salt, and pepper over the chickpeas, and toss again to distribute the seasonings.
4. Spread the chickpeas out in a single layer on the prepared baking sheet.
5. Roast in the preheated oven for 25-30 minutes, or until the chickpeas are golden brown and crispy. Shake the pan or stir the chickpeas halfway through to ensure even roasting.
6. Let the chickpeas cool before serving. They can be enjoyed warm or at room temperature as a crunchy, savory snack.

Walnut and Date Energy Balls

Ingredients:

- 1 cup walnuts
- 1 cup pitted dates
- 1/4 cup unsweetened cocoa powder

- 1 teaspoon vanilla extract
- A pinch of salt
- Optional: shredded coconut, sesame seeds, or additional cocoa powder for coating

Instructions:

1. In a food processor, combine the walnuts and pitted dates. Pulse until the mixture starts to come together and the nuts are finely chopped.
2. Add the cocoa powder, vanilla extract, and a pinch of salt to the nut and date mixture. Process until the mixture forms a sticky dough.
3. Take small amounts of the mixture and roll them into balls, about 1 inch in diameter. If the mixture is too sticky, wet your hands slightly before rolling.
4. Optional: Roll the energy balls in shredded coconut, sesame seeds, or cocoa powder to coat the outside.
5. Place the energy balls on a plate or tray and refrigerate for at least 30 minutes to set.
6. These energy balls can be stored in an airtight container in the refrigerator for up to a week or in the freezer for longer storage.

Cucumber Rounds Topped with Smoked Salmon and Cream Cheese

Ingredients:

- 1 large English cucumber
- 4 ounces smoked salmon, thinly sliced
- 1/2 cup cream cheese, softened
- Fresh dill for garnish
- Black pepper to taste
- Optional: capers or lemon zest for extra flavor

Instructions:

1. Wash the cucumber and slice it into 1/4-inch thick rounds. Pat the slices dry with a paper towel to remove excess moisture.

2. Spread a small amount of cream cheese on each cucumber round. The back of a small spoon or a butter knife works well for this.

3. Place a small piece of smoked salmon on top of the cream cheese on each cucumber slice.

4. Garnish each cucumber round with a sprig of fresh dill. If desired, add a few capers or a sprinkle of lemon zest on top for added flavor.

5. Season with a light sprinkle of black pepper to taste.

6. Arrange the cucumber rounds on a serving platter and serve immediately.

Baked Sweet Potato Fries with Rosemary

Ingredients:

- 2 large sweet potatoes, peeled and cut into fries
- 2 tablespoons olive oil
- 1 tablespoon fresh rosemary, finely chopped (or 1 teaspoon dried rosemary)
- Salt and pepper to taste

Instructions:

1. Preheat the oven to 425°F (220°C). Line a baking sheet with parchment paper for easy cleanup.
2. In a large bowl, toss the sweet potato fries with olive oil, ensuring each piece is well coated.
3. Sprinkle the chopped rosemary over the sweet potatoes, along with salt and pepper, and toss again to distribute the seasonings evenly.
4. Spread the sweet potato fries out in a single layer on the prepared baking sheet, making sure they're not overcrowded to ensure even cooking and crispiness.

5. Bake in the preheated oven for 25-30 minutes, or until the fries are tender on the inside and crispy on the outside. Flip the fries halfway through baking for even crispiness.

6. Serve the baked sweet potato fries hot, as a flavorful and nutritious side dish that pairs well with a variety of mains.

Steamed Edamame with Sea Salt

Ingredients:

- 2 cups frozen edamame in pods
- Sea salt to taste

Instructions:

1. Bring a pot of water to a boil. You can use a steamer basket if you have one; if not, you can place the edamame directly in the boiling water.

2. Add the frozen edamame to the pot and cover. If you're using a steamer basket, ensure it's suspended above the boiling water, not submerged.

3. Steam the edamame for about 5-6 minutes or until they are heated through and tender.

4. Drain the edamame and transfer them to a serving bowl.

5. Sprinkle generously with sea salt while they're still warm, tossing to ensure the pods are evenly coated.

6. Serve the steamed edamame as a snack or appetizer. Enjoy by squeezing the beans out of the pods directly into your mouth, and discarding the pods.

Kale Chips Baked

Ingredients:

- 1 large bunch of kale, stems removed and leaves torn into bite-sized pieces
- 1-2 tablespoons olive oil
- 2 tablespoons nutritional yeast
- Salt to taste

Instructions:

1. Preheat your oven to 300°F (150°C). Line a baking sheet with parchment paper.
2. Wash the kale leaves and dry them thoroughly. Any moisture will prevent the kale chips from becoming crispy.
3. In a large bowl, toss the kale leaves with olive oil, ensuring each leaf is lightly coated. Use your hands to massage the oil into the leaves for even coverage.
4. Sprinkle the nutritional yeast over the kale, along with a pinch of salt. Toss again to distribute the seasonings evenly.

5. Arrange the kale leaves in a single layer on the prepared baking sheet, making sure they don't overlap to ensure even baking and crispiness.

6. Bake in the preheated oven for 10-15 minutes, or until the edges are crispy but not burnt. Keep a close eye on them, as they can go from perfect to burnt quickly.

7. Let the kale chips cool on the baking sheet for a few minutes; they will crisp up further as they cool.

8. Serve the kale chips as a nutritious and flavorful snack that's perfect for satisfying crunchy cravings.

CHAPTER 6: Desserts

Baked Apples with Cinnamon and Walnuts

Ingredients:

- 4 large apples (such as Fuji or Gala)
- 1/2 cup walnuts, chopped
- 1/4 cup raisins or dried cranberries
- 2 tablespoons honey or maple syrup
- 1 teaspoon ground cinnamon
- 1/4 teaspoon ground nutmeg
- 1/2 cup apple juice or water
- Optional: A dollop of Greek yogurt for serving

Instructions:

1. Preheat the oven to 350°F (175°C).
2. Core the apples, leaving the bottom intact to create a well. If needed, slice a small amount off the bottom of each apple to ensure they sit flat in the baking dish.
3. In a small bowl, mix the chopped walnuts, raisins (or dried cranberries), honey (or maple syrup), cinnamon, and nutmeg.
4. Stuff each apple with the walnut mixture, packing it well into the hollowed-out core.

5. Place the stuffed apples in a baking dish. Pour the apple juice or water into the bottom of the dish around the apples.

6. Cover the dish with aluminum foil and bake for 20 minutes. Remove the foil and continue baking for an additional 20-25 minutes, or until the apples are tender but not mushy.

7. Serve the baked apples warm, with a dollop of Greek yogurt on top if desired, for an extra creamy contrast to the warm spices.

Blueberry Almond Chia Pudding

Ingredients:

- 1/4 cup chia seeds
- 1 cup unsweetened almond milk
- 1/2 teaspoon vanilla extract
- 1 tablespoon honey or maple syrup
- 1/2 cup fresh or frozen blueberries
- 2 tablespoons slivered almonds
- Optional: Additional honey or maple syrup for drizzling

Instructions:

1. In a bowl, combine the chia seeds, almond milk, vanilla extract, and honey (or maple syrup). Whisk together until well mixed.

2. Cover the bowl and refrigerate for at least 2 hours, or overnight, until the mixture thickens and achieves a pudding-like consistency.

3. Once the chia pudding is set, stir it well. If the pudding is too thick, you can add a little more almond milk to reach your desired consistency.

4. Layer the chia pudding in serving glasses or bowls with fresh or thawed blueberries and slivered almonds.

5. Drizzle with additional honey or maple syrup if a sweeter taste is desired.

6. Serve the blueberry almond chia pudding chilled as a nutritious and satisfying dessert or breakfast option.

Dark Chocolate-Dipped Strawberries

Ingredients:

- 1 pound fresh strawberries, washed and dried
- 6 ounces dark chocolate (at least 70% cocoa)
- 1 tablespoon coconut oil (optional, for smoother chocolate)
- Optional toppings: chopped nuts, shredded coconut, or cocoa powder

Instructions:

1. Line a baking sheet with parchment paper or a silicone baking mat.

2. In a microwave-safe bowl, break the dark chocolate into pieces and add the coconut oil. Microwave in 30-second intervals,

stirring in between, until the chocolate is completely melted and smooth. Be careful not to overheat.

3. Hold the strawberries by the stem and dip each one into the melted chocolate, twirling gently to let the excess chocolate drip off.

4. Place the dipped strawberries on the prepared baking sheet. If using any optional toppings, sprinkle them on the strawberries before the chocolate sets.

5. Refrigerate the strawberries for about 30 minutes, or until the chocolate has hardened.

6. Serve the chocolate-dipped strawberries.

Whole Wheat Banana Bread with Flaxseeds

Ingredients:

- 2 cups whole wheat flour
- 1/4 cup ground flaxseeds
- 1 teaspoon baking soda
- 1/2 teaspoon salt
- 1/2 cup unsalted butter, softened
- 3/4 cup honey or pure maple syrup
- 2 large eggs
- 1 1/2 cups mashed ripe bananas (about 3-4 bananas)
- 1/4 cup milk (dairy or plant-based)
- 1 teaspoon vanilla extract

- 1/2 cup walnuts, chopped (optional)

Instructions:

1. Preheat your oven to 350°F (175°C). Grease a 9x5 inch loaf pan or line it with parchment paper.
2. In a medium bowl, whisk together the whole wheat flour, ground flaxseeds, baking soda, and salt.
3. In a large bowl, beat the softened butter and honey (or maple syrup) with an electric mixer until well combined. Add the eggs one at a time, beating well after each addition.
4. Stir in the mashed bananas, milk, and vanilla extract until well blended.
5. Gradually add the dry ingredients to the wet ingredients, stirring just until the flour is incorporated. Avoid overmixing. Fold in the chopped walnuts if using.
6. Pour the batter into the prepared loaf pan and smooth the top with a spatula.
7. Bake in the preheated oven for 55-60 minutes, or until a toothpick inserted into the center comes out clean.
8. Let the banana bread cool in the pan for 10 minutes, then transfer it to a wire rack to cool completely.
9. Slice and serve the banana bread.

Mixed Berry and Yogurt Parfait

Ingredients:

- 2 cups Greek yogurt (plain or vanilla)
- 1 cup mixed berries (strawberries, blueberries, raspberries, blackberries)
- 1/2 cup granola
- 2 tablespoons honey or maple syrup (optional)
- A few mint leaves for garnish (optional)

Instructions:

1. If using strawberries, slice them into smaller pieces to match the size of the other berries.
2. In serving glasses or bowls, begin by layering a spoonful of Greek yogurt at the bottom.
3. Add a layer of mixed berries on top of the yogurt.
4. Sprinkle a layer of granola over the berries for a crunchy texture.
5. Repeat the layers until the glasses or bowls are filled, ending with a layer of berries on top for a visually appealing presentation.
6. Drizzle honey or maple syrup over the top layer if a sweeter taste is desired.
7. Garnish with a mint leaf on top of each parfait for a touch of freshness.

8. Serve the parfaits immediately or refrigerate them for up to an hour before serving to allow the flavors to meld together. Enjoy.

Almond and Date Energy Bites

Ingredients:

- 1 cup almonds
- 1 cup pitted dates
- 1/4 cup unsweetened shredded coconut
- 1 tablespoon chia seeds
- 1 teaspoon vanilla extract
- A pinch of salt

Instructions:

1. In a food processor, pulse the almonds until they are coarsely chopped. Be careful not to over-process; you want some texture for crunch.
2. Add the pitted dates to the food processor with the chopped almonds. Process until the mixture starts to stick together and forms a dough-like consistency.
3. Add the shredded coconut, chia seeds, vanilla extract, and a pinch of salt to the mixture. Pulse a few more times until all ingredients are well combined and the mixture is sticky.

4. Scoop out the mixture by tablespoons and roll it into balls between the palms of your hands. If the mixture is too sticky, wet your hands slightly with water to make rolling easier.

5. Place the formed energy bites on a baking sheet or large plate lined with parchment paper.

6. Refrigerate the energy bites for at least 30 minutes to firm up before serving.

7. Store the energy bites in an airtight container in the refrigerator for up to a week or in the freezer for longer storage. Enjoy.

Peach and Berry Cobbler with Oat Topping

Ingredients for Filling:

- 3 cups fresh or frozen peaches, sliced
- 2 cups mixed berries (such as blueberries, raspberries, and blackberries)
- 1/4 cup honey or maple syrup
- 1 tablespoon lemon juice
- 2 teaspoons cornstarch or arrowroot powder

Ingredients for Oat Topping:

- 1 cup rolled oats
- 1/2 cup whole wheat flour
- 1/3 cup brown sugar or coconut sugar
- 1/2 teaspoon ground cinnamon

- 1/4 cup unsalted butter, melted
- 1/4 cup chopped walnuts or almonds (optional)

Instructions:

1. Preheat your oven to 375°F (190°C). Grease a 9-inch baking dish.

2. In a large bowl, combine the sliced peaches, mixed berries, honey or maple syrup, lemon juice, and cornstarch. Toss gently to coat the fruit evenly. Transfer the fruit mixture to the prepared baking dish.

3. In another bowl, mix the rolled oats, whole wheat flour, brown sugar, and cinnamon. Pour the melted butter over the oat mixture and stir until the mixture resembles coarse crumbs. If using, stir in the chopped nuts.

4. Sprinkle the oat topping evenly over the fruit mixture in the baking dish.

5. Bake in the preheated oven for 35-40 minutes, or until the topping is golden brown and the fruit filling is bubbling around the edges.

6. Let the cobbler cool slightly before serving. Enjoy warm, perhaps with a dollop of Greek yogurt or a scoop of vanilla ice cream for an extra treat.

Avocado Chocolate Mousse

Ingredients:

- 2 ripe avocados, peeled and pitted
- 1/3 cup cocoa powder
- 1/4 cup honey or maple syrup (adjust to taste)
- 1/4 cup milk (dairy or plant-based)
- 1 teaspoon vanilla extract
- A pinch of salt
- Optional toppings: fresh berries, shredded coconut, or chopped nuts

Instructions:

1. In a food processor or blender, combine the avocados, cocoa powder, honey or maple syrup, milk, vanilla extract, and a pinch of salt.
2. Blend until the mixture is smooth and creamy, scraping down the sides as needed. Taste and adjust the sweetness if necessary.
3. Divide the mousse into serving dishes and refrigerate for at least 30 minutes to chill and set.
4. Before serving, garnish the avocado chocolate mousse with your choice of toppings such as fresh berries, shredded coconut, or chopped nuts.

Carrot Cake Muffins with Whole Wheat Flour

Ingredients:

- 1 1/2 cups whole wheat flour
- 1 teaspoon baking soda
- 1/2 teaspoon salt
- 1 teaspoon ground cinnamon
- 1/2 teaspoon ground nutmeg
- 1/2 cup unsweetened applesauce
- 1/4 cup olive oil or melted coconut oil
- 1/2 cup honey or maple syrup
- 2 eggs
- 1 teaspoon vanilla extract
- 1 1/2 cups grated carrots (about 2-3 medium carrots)
- 1/2 cup chopped walnuts or pecans (optional)
- 1/4 cup raisins (optional)

Instructions:

1. Preheat your oven to 350°F (175°C). Line a muffin tin with paper liners or grease with oil.
2. In a large bowl, whisk together the whole wheat flour, baking soda, salt, cinnamon, and nutmeg.

3. In a separate bowl, mix the applesauce, oil, honey, eggs, and vanilla extract until well combined.

4. Pour the wet ingredients into the dry ingredients and stir until just combined. Be careful not to overmix.

5. Fold in the grated carrots, and if using, the chopped nuts and raisins.

6. Divide the batter evenly among the muffin cups, filling each about 3/4 full.

7. Bake for 18-22 minutes, or until a toothpick inserted into the center of a muffin comes out clean.

8. Let the muffins cool in the tin for a few minutes, then transfer to a wire rack to cool completely.

9. Serve these wholesome carrot cake muffins as a nutritious breakfast or snack, enjoying the natural sweetness and moisture from the carrots and applesauce.

Grilled Pineapple with Honey and Greek Yogurt

Ingredients:

- 1 fresh pineapple, peeled, cored, and cut into rings or wedges
- 2 tablespoons honey
- 1 cup Greek yogurt
- A pinch of ground cinnamon or nutmeg (optional)
- Fresh mint leaves for garnish (optional)

Instructions:

1. Preheat a grill or grill pan over medium heat.

2. Brush the pineapple rings or wedges lightly with honey on both sides.

3. Place the pineapple on the grill and cook for 2-3 minutes per side, or until the pineapple has nice grill marks and is slightly caramelized.

4. Remove the pineapple from the grill and allow it to cool slightly.

5. Serve the grilled pineapple with a dollop of Greek yogurt on the side or top of each pineapple piece.

6. Drizzle with a little more honey and sprinkle with a pinch of cinnamon or nutmeg if desired.

7. Garnish with fresh mint leaves for a refreshing touch.

CHAPTER 7: Smoothies and Beverages

Blueberry Walnut Smoothie

Ingredients:

- 1 cup blueberries (fresh or frozen)
- 1/4 cup walnuts
- 1 cup spinach leaves (fresh)
- 1 banana, peeled
- 1 cup almond milk (unsweetened)

Instructions:

1. In a blender, combine the blueberries, walnuts, spinach, banana, and almond milk.
2. Blend on high until the mixture is smooth and creamy. If the smoothie is too thick, you can add a little more almond milk to reach your desired consistency.
3. Taste and adjust the sweetness, if necessary, by adding a teaspoon of honey or maple syrup and blending again.
4. Pour the smoothie into a glass and enjoy immediately.

Strawberry Oat Heart-Healthy Smoothie

Ingredients:

- 1 cup strawberries (fresh or frozen)

- 1/4 cup rolled oats
- 1 tablespoon flaxseeds
- 1 cup Greek yogurt (plain, unsweetened)
- Honey or maple syrup to taste (optional)

Instructions:

1. Place the strawberries, rolled oats, and flaxseeds in a blender. If you're using frozen strawberries, there's no need to thaw them first as they'll help make the smoothie cold and thick.

2. Add the Greek yogurt to the blender. Greek yogurt adds a creamy texture and a good dose of protein.

3. Blend on high until the ingredients are thoroughly combined and the mixture is smooth. Depending on the power of your blender, you may need to stop and stir the ingredients a few times or add a splash of milk or water to help everything blend smoothly.

4. Taste the smoothie and add a bit of honey or maple syrup if you prefer it sweeter. Blend again to mix through.

5. Serve the smoothie in a tall glass.

Green Tea and Citrus Boost

Ingredients:

- 1 cup brewed green tea, cooled
- Juice of 1 orange
- Juice of 1/2 a lemon

- 1/2 cup fresh spinach leaves
- 1 tablespoon honey (optional)
- Ice cubes

Instructions:

1. Brew a cup of green tea and allow it to cool to room temperature or chill it in the refrigerator.
2. In a blender, combine the cooled green tea, orange juice, lemon juice, and fresh spinach leaves.
3. Add honey if you prefer a sweeter taste.
4. Add a handful of ice cubes to the blender.
5. Blend all the ingredients until smooth and well combined.
6. Pour the smoothie into a glass and enjoy immediately.

Turmeric Ginger Zinger

Ingredients:

- 1-inch fresh turmeric root, peeled and chopped (or 1 teaspoon turmeric powder)
- 1-inch fresh ginger root, peeled and chopped
- 1 cup carrot juice (preferably freshly juiced)
- Juice of 1/2 a lemon
- A pinch of black pepper (to enhance turmeric absorption)
- Honey to taste (optional)
- Ice cubes

Instructions:

1. If using fresh turmeric and ginger roots, start by peeling and roughly chopping them.

2. In a blender, combine the chopped turmeric, ginger, carrot juice, and lemon juice.

3. Add a pinch of black pepper. This is important as it helps enhance the absorption of curcumin, the active compound in turmeric.

4. If you like your beverage a bit sweeter, add honey to taste.

5. Add a few ice cubes to the blender if you prefer your drink chilled.

6. Blend all the ingredients until smooth. If your blender struggles with the fibrous nature of turmeric and ginger, you may strain the drink through a fine mesh sieve or cheesecloth.

7. Serve the zinger immediately.

Avocado and Kale Smoothie

Ingredients:

- 1/2 ripe avocado
- 1 cup kale leaves, stems removed
- 1/2 green apple, cored and sliced
- 1 tablespoon chia seeds
- 1 cup coconut water or almond milk
- Ice cubes (optional for a colder smoothie)

- Honey or maple syrup to taste (optional)

Instructions:

1. In a blender, combine the avocado, kale leaves, green apple slices, and chia seeds.
2. Add the coconut water or almond milk to facilitate blending. If you prefer a colder smoothie, add a few ice cubes.
3. Blend on high until the mixture becomes smooth and creamy.
4. Taste the smoothie and, if desired, add a little honey or maple syrup for sweetness. Blend again to mix well.
5. Pour the smoothie into a glass and enjoy immediately.

Berry and Beet Detox Smoothie

Ingredients:

- 1/2 cooked beet, peeled and chopped
- 1 cup mixed berries (such as strawberries, blueberries, raspberries)
- 1 tablespoon ground flaxseed
- 1 cup spinach leaves
- 1 cup unsweetened almond milk or water
- Ice cubes (optional)
- Honey or maple syrup to taste (optional)

Instructions:

1. If not using pre-cooked beets, boil or roast a beet until tender, then cool, peel, and chop.

2. In a blender, add the chopped beet, mixed berries, ground flaxseed, and spinach leaves.

3. Pour in the almond milk or water for the liquid. Add ice cubes if you prefer a chilled smoothie.

4. Blend all the ingredients on high until the smoothie reaches a smooth consistency.

5. Taste and adjust the sweetness by adding honey or maple syrup if needed. Blend again to incorporate the sweetener.

6. Serve the smoothie immediately.

Almond Butter and Banana Protein Shake

Ingredients:

- 1 ripe banana
- 2 tablespoons almond butter
- 1 cup unsweetened almond milk
- 1 scoop plant-based protein powder (optional)
- A dash of cinnamon
- Ice cubes (optional)

Instructions:

1. Peel the banana and break it into chunks.

2. Place the banana chunks, almond butter, almond milk, and protein powder (if using) into a blender.

3. Add a dash of cinnamon for flavor. If you like your shake cold, add a few ice cubes.

4. Blend on high until the mixture is smooth and creamy.

5. Pour the shake into a glass and enjoy immediately.

Pomegranate and Cherry Antioxidant Drink

Ingredients:

- 1/2 cup pomegranate juice (freshly squeezed if possible)
- 1/2 cup cherry juice (unsweetened)
- 1 cup sparkling water
- Ice cubes
- Fresh mint leaves for garnish (optional)

Instructions:

1. In a large glass, combine the pomegranate juice and cherry juice. Both juices are known for their high antioxidant content.

2. Add the sparkling water to the juice mixture, creating a fizzy, refreshing beverage.

3. Add ice cubes to the glass to chill the drink.

4. Garnish with fresh mint leaves, if desired, for an added refreshing flavor.

5. Stir gently before serving.

Cucumber Mint Refresh

Ingredients:

- 1 large cucumber, peeled and roughly chopped
- Juice of 1 lime
- A handful of fresh mint leaves
- 1 cup cold water
- Ice cubes
- Honey or agave syrup to taste (optional)

Instructions:

1. Place the chopped cucumber, lime juice, mint leaves, and cold water into a blender.
2. Blend until smooth. For a sweeter drink, add honey or agave syrup to taste and blend again.
3. Strain the mixture through a fine mesh sieve or cheesecloth into a pitcher to remove the pulp and mint leaves, pressing to extract as much liquid as possible.
4. Serve the refreshment over ice cubes in glasses. Garnish with additional mint leaves or thin cucumber slices if desired.
5. Enjoy this cooling and hydrating drink, perfect for warm days or as a refreshing detox beverage.

Golden Milk Latte

Ingredients:

- 1 cup almond milk (or any milk of your choice)
- 1 teaspoon turmeric powder
- 1/2 teaspoon cinnamon powder
- 1/4 teaspoon ginger powder (or 1/2 inch fresh ginger, grated)
- A pinch of black pepper (to enhance turmeric absorption)
- 1 teaspoon honey or maple syrup (adjust to taste)
- 1/2 teaspoon vanilla extract (optional)

Instructions:

1. In a small saucepan, combine the almond milk, turmeric powder, cinnamon, ginger, and a pinch of black pepper. If using fresh ginger, add it to the pan as well.

2. Warm the mixture over medium heat, stirring constantly to prevent lumps and ensure even mixing of the spices. Do not let it boil.

3. Once the mixture is hot and steaming, remove it from the heat. If you use fresh ginger, strain the latte to remove the pieces.

4. Stir in the honey (or maple syrup) and vanilla extract if using, mixing well until dissolved.

5. Pour the golden milk latte into a mug. You can use a milk frother to froth the top if desired. Sprinkle a little extra cinnamon on top for garnish and enjoy warm.

CHAPTER 8: SOUPS

Lentil and Vegetable Soup

Ingredients:

- 1 cup dried green or brown lentils, rinsed and drained
- 2 tablespoons olive oil
- 1 onion, diced
- 2 carrots, peeled and diced
- 2 celery stalks, diced
- 2 garlic cloves, minced
- 1 teaspoon dried thyme
- 1 bay leaf
- 4 cups vegetable broth
- 2 cups water
- 1 can (14 oz) diced tomatoes, with juice
- 2 cups chopped kale or spinach
- Salt and pepper to taste
- Lemon wedges for serving (optional)

Instructions:

1. Heat olive oil in a large pot over medium heat. Add onion, carrots, and celery, and sauté until the vegetables start to soften, about 5 minutes.

2. Add garlic, thyme, and bay leaf, and cook for another minute until fragrant.

3. Stir in the lentils, vegetable broth, water, and diced tomatoes with their juice. Season with salt and pepper.

4. Bring the soup to a boil, then reduce the heat to low, cover, and simmer for about 30 minutes, or until the lentils are tender.

5. Add the chopped kale or spinach to the pot and cook for an additional 5 minutes, or until the greens are wilted and tender.

6. Remove the bay leaf and adjust the seasoning if necessary.

7. Serve the soup hot, with lemon wedges on the side for a refreshing squeeze of lemon juice if desired.

Tomato Basil Soup with Whole whole-grain croutons

Ingredients for Soup:

- 2 tablespoons olive oil
- 1 onion, diced
- 2 garlic cloves, minced
- 1 can (28 oz) whole peeled tomatoes, with juice
- 2 cups vegetable broth
- 1/4 cup fresh basil leaves, plus more for garnish
- Salt and pepper to taste
- 1/4 cup heavy cream or coconut milk (optional, for creaminess)

Ingredients for Whole Grain Croutons:

- 2 slices whole grain bread, cubed
- 1 tablespoon olive oil
- 1/2 teaspoon garlic powder
- Salt to taste

Instructions for Soup:

1. Heat olive oil in a large pot over medium heat. Add onion and cook until translucent, about 5 minutes. Add garlic and cook for another minute until fragrant.
2. Add the whole peeled tomatoes with their juice and vegetable broth. Bring to a simmer, breaking up the tomatoes with a spoon.
3. Add the basil leaves and season with salt and pepper. Simmer for 20 minutes.
4. Use an immersion blender to puree the soup until smooth. If desired, stir in heavy cream or coconut milk for a creamier texture.
5. Adjust seasoning if necessary.

Instructions for Whole Grain Croutons:

6. Preheat the oven to 375°F (190°C). Toss the cubed whole-grain bread with olive oil, garlic powder, and salt.

7. Spread the bread cubes in a single layer on a baking sheet. Bake until crispy and golden, about 10-15 minutes, stirring halfway through.

8. Serve the tomato basil soup hot, garnished with fresh basil leaves, and topped with homemade whole-grain croutons.

White Bean and Kale Minestrone

Ingredients:

- 2 tablespoons olive oil
- 1 onion, chopped
- 2 carrots, peeled and diced
- 2 celery stalks, diced
- 3 garlic cloves, minced
- 1 can (14 oz) diced tomatoes, with juice
- 4 cups vegetable broth
- 2 cups water
- 1 can (15 oz) white beans (such as cannellini or Great Northern), rinsed and drained
- 1 teaspoon dried oregano
- 1 teaspoon dried basil
- 1 bay leaf
- 2 cups kale, stems removed and leaves torn into bite-sized pieces
- 1 cup small pasta shapes (whole wheat or other whole grains preferred)

- Salt and pepper to taste
- Grated Parmesan cheese for serving (optional)

Instructions:

1. Heat olive oil in a large pot over medium heat. Add the onion, carrots, and celery, and sauté until the vegetables are softened, about 5 minutes.
2. Add the garlic and cook for another minute until fragrant.
3. Stir in the diced tomatoes with their juice, vegetable broth, water, white beans, oregano, basil, and bay leaf. Season with salt and pepper to taste.
4. Bring the soup to a boil, then reduce the heat and simmer for about 15 minutes.
5. Add the kale and pasta to the pot, and continue to simmer until the pasta is cooked and the kale is tender, about 10 minutes.
6. Remove the bay leaf and adjust the seasoning if necessary.
7. Serve the minestrone hot, sprinkled with grated Parmesan cheese if desired.

Carrot Ginger Soup with Turmeric

Ingredients:

- 2 tablespoons olive oil
- 1 onion, diced
- 1 pound carrots, peeled and chopped

- 2 tablespoons fresh ginger, minced
- 1 teaspoon turmeric powder
- 4 cups vegetable broth
- Salt and pepper to taste
- 1 can (14 oz) coconut milk
- Fresh cilantro for garnish (optional)

Instructions:

1. Heat olive oil in a large pot over medium heat. Add the onion and cook until translucent, about 5 minutes.
2. Add the chopped carrots and minced ginger to the pot. Cook for another 5 minutes, stirring occasionally.
3. Stir in the turmeric powder, and cook for 1 minute until fragrant.
4. Add the vegetable broth to the pot. Season with salt and pepper. Bring the mixture to a boil, then reduce the heat and simmer, covered, until the carrots are tender, about 20 minutes.
5. Use an immersion blender to puree the soup until smooth. Alternatively, you can carefully transfer the soup to a blender to puree in batches.
6. Stir in the coconut milk until well combined and heated through.
7. Adjust the seasoning if necessary.
8. Serve the soup hot, garnished with fresh cilantro if desired.

Quinoa and Black Bean Chili

Ingredients:

- 1 tablespoon olive oil
- 1 onion, diced
- 2 garlic cloves, minced
- 1 bell pepper, diced
- 1 jalapeño, seeded and minced (optional)
- 1 cup quinoa, rinsed
- 1 can (15 oz) black beans, drained and rinsed
- 1 can (14 oz) diced tomatoes, with juice
- 3 cups vegetable broth
- 2 tablespoons chili powder
- 1 tablespoon cumin
- Salt and pepper to taste
- Optional toppings: diced avocado, chopped cilantro, lime wedges, shredded cheese

Instructions:

1. Heat olive oil in a large pot over medium heat. Add the onion, garlic, bell pepper, and jalapeño (if using). Sauté until the vegetables are softened, about 5 minutes.
2. Stir in the quinoa, black beans, diced tomatoes, vegetable broth, chili powder, and cumin. Season with salt and pepper.

3. Bring the chili to a boil, then reduce the heat, cover, and simmer for about 25-30 minutes, or until the quinoa is cooked and the chili has thickened.

4. Taste and adjust seasoning as needed.

5. Serve the chili hot, with optional toppings like diced avocado, chopped cilantro, lime wedges, or shredded cheese.

Mushroom Barley Soup

Ingredients:

- 1 tablespoon olive oil
- 1 onion, chopped
- 2 carrots, diced
- 2 celery stalks, diced
- 3 garlic cloves, minced
- 1 pound of mushrooms, sliced (a mix of varieties works well)
- 3/4 cup pearl barley, rinsed
- 6 cups vegetable broth
- 1 teaspoon dried thyme
- Salt and pepper to taste
- Fresh parsley for garnish

Instructions:

1. Heat olive oil in a large pot over medium heat.

2. Add the onion, carrots, celery, and garlic. Sauté until the vegetables start to soften, about 5 minutes.

3. Add the sliced mushrooms to the pot and cook until they release their moisture and begin to brown about 8-10 minutes.

4. Stir in the pearl barley, vegetable broth, and dried thyme. Season with salt and pepper.

5. Bring the soup to a boil, then reduce the heat, cover, and simmer for about 45 minutes, or until the barley is tender and the soup has thickened.

6. Taste and adjust seasoning as needed.

7. Serve the soup hot, garnished with fresh parsley.

Split Pea Soup with Thyme

Ingredients:

- 1 cup dried split peas, rinsed and sorted
- 2 tablespoons olive oil
- 1 large onion, diced
- 2 carrots, peeled and diced
- 2 celery stalks, diced
- 2 garlic cloves, minced
- 1 teaspoon dried thyme
- 6 cups vegetable broth
- 1 bay leaf
- Salt and pepper to taste

- Optional: diced ham or smoked paprika for a smoky flavor

Instructions:

1. In a large pot, heat the olive oil over medium heat. Add the onion, carrots, and celery. Sauté until the vegetables are softened, about 5 minutes.
2. Add the minced garlic and dried thyme, and cook for another minute until fragrant.
3. Stir in the rinsed split peas, vegetable broth, and bay leaf. Season with salt and pepper. If using, add diced ham or a sprinkle of smoked paprika for a smoky flavor.
4. Bring the soup to a boil, then reduce the heat to low. Cover and simmer for 60-90 minutes, or until the split peas are soft and the soup has thickened. Stir occasionally to prevent sticking.
5. Remove the bay leaf and adjust the seasoning as needed. For a smoother soup, you can use an immersion blender to puree part of the soup.
6. Serve hot, enjoying the hearty and comforting flavors.

Butternut Squash and Apple Soup

Ingredients:

- 1 medium butternut squash, peeled, seeded, and cubed
- 2 tablespoons olive oil
- 1 onion, diced

- 2 apples, peeled, cored, and chopped (tart varieties work well)
- 1 teaspoon ground cinnamon
- 1/2 teaspoon ground nutmeg
- 4 cups vegetable broth
- Salt and pepper to taste
- Optional garnishes: a swirl of cream, toasted pumpkin seeds, or fresh thyme leaves

Instructions:

1. In a large pot, heat the olive oil over medium heat. Add the diced onion and cook until translucent, about 5 minutes.
2. Add the cubed butternut squash and chopped apples to the pot. Cook for another 5-7 minutes, until the apples begin to soften.
3. Stir in the ground cinnamon and nutmeg, coating the squash and apples evenly.
4. Pour in the vegetable broth and season with salt and pepper. Bring the mixture to a boil, then reduce the heat, cover, and simmer for 20-30 minutes, or until the butternut squash is tender.
5. Use an immersion blender to puree the soup until smooth. Alternatively, you can carefully transfer the soup to a blender and puree in batches.
6. Taste and adjust seasoning as needed. Serve the soup hot, garnished with your choice of cream, toasted pumpkin seeds, or fresh thyme leaves for added flavor and texture.

Broccoli Almond Soup

Ingredients:

- 2 tablespoons olive oil
- 1 onion, diced
- 2 garlic cloves, minced
- 4 cups broccoli florets
- 1/3 cup raw almonds, plus more for garnish
- 4 cups vegetable broth
- Salt and pepper to taste
- A pinch of nutmeg (optional)
- Lemon juice to taste (optional)

Instructions:

1. Heat olive oil in a large pot over medium heat. Add the diced onion and cook until translucent, about 5 minutes.
2. Add the minced garlic and cook for an additional minute until fragrant.
3. Add the broccoli florets and raw almonds to the pot, stirring to combine.
4. Pour in the vegetable broth, and season with salt, pepper, and a pinch of nutmeg if using. Bring the mixture to a boil.
5. Reduce the heat to low, cover, and simmer for 20-25 minutes, or until the broccoli is tender and the almonds are softened.

6. Use an immersion blender to puree the soup until smooth. Alternatively, you can carefully transfer the soup to a blender and puree in batches. Be cautious as the soup will be hot.

7. Taste and adjust the seasoning as needed, adding a splash of lemon juice for a bit of acidity if desired.

8. Serve the soup hot, garnished with chopped almonds for added crunch.

Chickpea and Spinach Stew

Ingredients:

- 2 tablespoons olive oil
- 1 onion, diced
- 3 garlic cloves, minced
- 1 teaspoon ground cumin
- 1/2 teaspoon smoked paprika
- 1 can (15 oz) chickpeas, drained and rinsed
- 1 can (14 oz) diced tomatoes, with juice
- 4 cups fresh spinach leaves
- 3 cups vegetable broth
- Salt and pepper to taste
- Lemon wedges for serving (optional)

Instructions:

1. Heat olive oil in a large pot over medium heat.

2. Add the diced onion and cook until softened about 5 minutes.

3. Add the minced garlic, ground cumin, and smoked paprika to the pot. Cook for another minute until the spices are fragrant.

4. Stir in the chickpeas and diced tomatoes with their juice. Cook for a few minutes to allow the flavors to meld.

5. Add the vegetable broth to the pot and bring the mixture to a simmer.

6. Gradually add the spinach leaves, stirring until they wilt into the stew.

7. Season the stew with salt and pepper to taste. Simmer for an additional 10-15 minutes to allow the flavors to deepen.

8. Serve the stew hot, with lemon wedges on the side for squeezing over the top if desired.

CONCLUSION

In crafting this MIND diet cookbook for seniors over 60, we've journeyed through a collection of recipes designed not only to nourish the body but also to protect and enhance cognitive function. Each recipe, from the nutrient-rich smoothies to the hearty soups and stews, and from the vibrant salads to the comforting desserts, has been tailored with seniors' specific nutritional needs and taste preferences in mind.

The MIND diet, a fusion of the Mediterranean and DASH diets, emphasizes foods known to benefit brain health, such as leafy greens, berries, whole grains, and lean proteins. This cookbook aims to make these dietary principles accessible and enjoyable, offering a variety of flavors and ingredients to cater to diverse palates and dietary requirements.

By incorporating these recipes into their daily lives, seniors can enjoy meals that not only delight the senses but also contribute to a healthy, vibrant lifestyle that supports brain health. The hope is that this cookbook will serve not just as a guide for preparing meals but also as a tool for empowering seniors to take an active role in maintaining their cognitive well-being through nutrition.

Let this cookbook be a testament to the joy of cooking and eating well at any age, with the added benefit of supporting a sharp and active mind.

28-DAY MEAL PLAN

Day 1:

Breakfast: Blueberry Almond Oatmeal

Lunch: Mediterranean Quinoa Salad

Dinner: Baked Cod with Lemon and Dill over Quinoa

Snack: Carrot and Celery Sticks with Hummus

Beverage: Cucumber Mint Refresh

Day 2:

Breakfast: Spinach and Feta Omelet

Lunch: Lentil Soup with Whole Grain Bread

Dinner: Roasted Chicken with Sweet Potatoes and Brussels Sprouts

Snack: Greek Yogurt with Blueberries and a Drizzle of Honey

Beverage: Green Tea and Citrus Boost

Day 3:

Breakfast: Avocado Toast with Poached Egg

Lunch: Turkey and Avocado Wrap

Dinner: Vegetable Lentil Stew with Whole Grain Rolls

Snack: Sliced Apple with Almond Butter

Beverage: Turmeric Ginger Zinger

Day 4:

Breakfast: Whole Grain Waffles with Mixed Berries

Lunch: Spinach and Strawberry Salad with Walnuts

Dinner: Grilled Vegetable and Bean Tacos with Avocado Salsa

Snack: Whole Grain Crackers with Avocado Mash

Beverage: Strawberry Oat Heart-Healthy Smoothie

Day 5:

Breakfast: Greek Yogurt Parfait

Lunch: Baked Sweet Potato with Black Bean Salsa

Dinner: Whole Wheat Pasta Primavera with Seasonal Vegetables

Snack: Roasted Chickpeas with Garlic and Herbs

Beverage: Blueberry Walnut Smoothie

Day 6:

Breakfast: Vegetable Frittata

Lunch: Broccoli and Almond Stir-Fry

Dinner: Stuffed Bell Peppers with Brown Rice and Turkey

Snack: Walnut and Date Energy Balls

Beverage: Almond Butter and Banana Protein Shake

Day 7:

Breakfast: Nutty Banana Smoothie

Lunch: Tuna Salad Stuffed Tomatoes

Dinner: Baked Eggplant Parmesan with a Side Salad

Snack: Cucumber Rounds Topped with Smoked Salmon and
Cream Cheese

Beverage: Pomegranate and Cherry Antioxidant Drink

Day 8:

Breakfast: Quinoa Breakfast Bowl

Lunch: Roasted Vegetable and Hummus Pita Pockets

Dinner: Salmon Quinoa Patties with Steamed Asparagus

Snack: Baked Sweet Potato Fries with Rosemary

Beverage: Golden Milk Latte

Day 9:

Breakfast: Kale and Mushroom Breakfast Sauté

Lunch: Barley and Roasted Beet Salad

Dinner: Turkey Meatballs in Tomato Sauce with Steamed Broccoli

Snack: Steamed Edamame with Sea Salt

Beverage: Avocado and Kale Smoothie

Day 10:

Breakfast: Blueberry Almond Oatmeal

Lunch: Grilled Salmon with Steamed Greens

Dinner: Spinach and Mushroom Stuffed Chicken Breast with Wild Rice

Snack: Kale Chips Baked with Olive Oil and Nutritional Yeast

Beverage: Berry and Beet Detox Smoothie

Day 11:

Breakfast: Spinach and Feta Omelet

Lunch: Lentil Soup with Whole Grain Bread

Dinner: Vegetable Lentil Stew with Whole Grain Rolls

Snack: Carrot and Celery Sticks with Hummus

Beverage: Cucumber Mint Refresh

Day 12:

Breakfast: Avocado Toast with Poached Egg

Lunch: Mediterranean Quinoa Salad

Dinner: Whole Wheat Pasta Primavera with Seasonal Vegetables

Snack: Greek Yogurt with Blueberries and a Drizzle of Honey

Beverage: Green Tea and Citrus Boost

Day 13:

Breakfast: Whole Grain Waffles with Mixed Berries

Lunch: Turkey and Avocado Wrap

Dinner: Baked Cod with Lemon and Dill over Quinoa

Snack: Sliced Apple with Almond Butter

Beverage: Turmeric Ginger Zinger

Day 14:

Breakfast: Greek Yogurt Parfait

Lunch: Spinach and Strawberry Salad with Walnuts

Dinner: Roasted Chicken with Sweet Potatoes and Brussels Sprouts

Snack: Whole Grain Crackers with Avocado Mash

Beverage: Strawberry Oat Heart-Healthy Smoothie

Day 15:

Breakfast: Nutty Banana Smoothie

Lunch: Baked Sweet Potato with Black Bean Salsa

Dinner: Grilled Vegetable and Bean Tacos with Avocado Salsa

Snack: Roasted Chickpeas with Garlic and Herbs

Beverage: Blueberry Walnut Smoothie

Day 16:

Breakfast: Vegetable Frittata

Lunch: Broccoli and Almond Stir-Fry

Dinner: Stuffed Bell Peppers with Brown Rice and Turkey

Snack: Walnut and Date Energy Balls

Beverage: Almond Butter and Banana Protein Shake

Day 17:

Breakfast: Quinoa Breakfast Bowl

Lunch: Tuna Salad Stuffed Tomatoes

Dinner: Baked Eggplant Parmesan with a Side Salad

Snack: Cucumber Rounds Topped with Smoked Salmon and Cream Cheese

Beverage: Pomegranate and Cherry Antioxidant Drink

Day 18:

Breakfast: Kale and Mushroom Breakfast Sauté

Lunch: Barley and Roasted Beet Salad

Dinner: Salmon Quinoa Patties with Steamed Asparagus

Snack: Baked Sweet Potato Fries with Rosemary

Beverage: Golden Milk Latte

Day 19:

Breakfast: Blueberry Almond Oatmeal

Lunch: Mediterranean Quinoa Salad

Dinner: Turkey Meatballs in Tomato Sauce with Steamed Broccoli

Snack: Steamed Edamame with Sea Salt

Beverage: Avocado and Kale Smoothie

Day 20:

Breakfast: Spinach and Feta Omelet

Lunch: Lentil Soup with Whole Grain Bread

Dinner: Vegetable Lentil Stew with Whole Grain Rolls

Snack: Kale Chips Baked with Olive Oil and Nutritional Yeast

Beverage: Berry and Beet Detox Smoothie

Day 21:

Breakfast: Avocado Toast with Poached Egg

Lunch: Grilled Salmon with Steamed Greens

Dinner: Whole Wheat Pasta Primavera with Seasonal Vegetables

Snack: Carrot and Celery Sticks with Hummus

Beverage: Cucumber Mint Refresh

Day 22:

Breakfast: Whole Grain Waffles with Mixed Berries

Lunch: Roasted Vegetable and Hummus Pita Pockets

Dinner: Baked Cod with Lemon and Dill over Quinoa

Snack: Greek Yogurt with Blueberries and a Drizzle of Honey

Beverage: Green Tea and Citrus Boost

Day 23:

Breakfast: Greek Yogurt Parfait

Lunch: Spinach and Strawberry Salad with Walnuts

Dinner: Roasted Chicken with Sweet Potatoes and Brussels Sprouts

Snack: Sliced Apple with Almond Butter

Beverage: Turmeric Ginger Zinger

Day 24:

Breakfast: Nutty Banana Smoothie

Lunch: Turkey and Avocado Wrap

Dinner: Grilled Vegetable and Bean Tacos with Avocado Salsa

Snack: Whole Grain Crackers with Avocado Mash

Beverage: Strawberry Oat Heart-Healthy Smoothie

Day 25:

Breakfast: Vegetable Frittata

Lunch: Baked Sweet Potato with Black Bean Salsa

Dinner: Stuffed Bell Peppers with Brown Rice and Turkey

Snack: Roasted Chickpeas with Garlic and Herbs

Beverage: Blueberry Walnut Smoothie

Day 26:

Breakfast: Quinoa Breakfast Bowl

Lunch: Broccoli and Almond Stir-Fry

Dinner: Whole Wheat Pasta Primavera with Seasonal Vegetables

Snack: Walnut and Date Energy Balls

Beverage: Almond Butter and Banana Protein Shake

Day 27:

Breakfast: Kale and Mushroom Breakfast Sauté

Lunch: Tuna Salad Stuffed Tomatoes

Dinner: Baked Eggplant Parmesan with a Side Salad

Snack: Cucumber Rounds Topped with Smoked Salmon and Cream Cheese

Beverage: Pomegranate and Cherry Antioxidant Drink

Day 28:

Breakfast: Blueberry Almond Oatmeal

Lunch: Mediterranean Quinoa Salad

Dinner: Salmon Quinoa Patties with Steamed Asparagus

Snack: Baked Sweet Potato Fries with Rosemary

Beverage: Golden Milk Latte

Weekly Shopping List

NO.	ITEM LIST	QUANTITY

NOTES

-
-
-

Weekly Shopping List

NO.	ITEM LIST	QUANTITY

NOTES

-
-
-

Weekly Shopping List

NO.	ITEM LIST	QUANTITY

NOTES

-
-
-

Weekly Shopping List

NO.	ITEM LIST	QUANTITY

NOTES
•
•
•

Weekly Shopping List

NO.	ITEM LIST	QUANTITY

NOTES

-
-
-

Weekly Shopping List

NO.	ITEM LIST	QUANTITY

NOTES
•
•
•

Weekly Shopping List

NO.	ITEM LIST	QUANTITY

NOTES

-
-
-

www.ingramcontent.com/pod-product-compliance
Lightning Source LLC
Chambersburg PA
CBHW071050290526
45795CB00004B/1417